The Body Whispers Before It Screams

*Facing Menopause
Physically, Emotionally,
and Spiritually*

IRENE ORTIZ-GLASS

Published by You Are Not Your Scars™ Publishing
Nashville, Tennessee

Cover and interior design by Chelsea Jewell

ISBN: 978-1-956822-02-1 Paperback
978-1-956822-03-8 eBook

Printed in the USA, Canada, Australia, and Europe

This book is dedicated to every woman suffering in silence. It's for every woman who feels like giving up because there is nobody who understands the struggle she is facing as her body and brain become unrecognizable. It's for every woman who deserves to thrive and find joy again.

I was you, I see you, there is hope in these pages.

—Irene Ortiz-Glass

Contents

Introduction

The weakness that overcame my mind and body was torture. What was supposed to be a normal transition in life was killing me.

My Wilderness was very dark and thick with moss. My feet felt stuck in the murky mud, and I had no idea what could lurk behind the trees. I was alone, unable to articulate how bad I felt, and terrified. The anxiety came in waves and rattled me to my core. My thoughts were uncontrollable and filled with ruminations. My body was unable to cope with any stress at all as the heat came up from my feet to the crown of my head. My focus was nonexistent as I struggled to work, which left me feeling defeated. This was my journey through perimenopause and surgical menopause.

I had seen so many doctors and had so many tests done. Most said, "This is normal" and "You just have to go through it." Others did their best to work in areas of their specialty, but nobody seemed able to "fix" me. I was broken and becoming smaller each day as I struggled to find energy to live. Why didn't anyone fully understand this? Why was it so hard? How could God let this happen to me? I had lost faith in the medical system, and it was clear that if I wanted to get better, I was going to have to go to battle. I just couldn't find the strength.

As the sun shone down on my face during a walk to calm my spirit, I poured my soul out to God. I cried aloud as I begged Him to tell me why I suffered. As if someone cracked open my soul, I felt His response so clearly. "You are asking the wrong question. You should be asking 'What?'" The word "*what*" turned over and over in my mind. God expected me to do something with all the struggle. I went home and started dumping everything that swirled in my mind on pages. I went back to my ten years of labs and thousands of pages of data. I prayed over the pages and asked God to bring me out of the abyss, to find my way home, to the person He created me to be. I knew God already, but through my struggles of perimenopause and then surgical menopause, I met Him in the most intimate way possible. Broken, weak, and exhausted, I made a commitment to find the "what."

This book is the "what." It is my story. It is about how I became an educated advocate and fought my way back. It's a miracle story, a comeback story, a story of resilience, faith, and surrender. It's about how to unravel all the lies you have been told about your health. It's about learning about your own body and its needs. And it's about reawakening your spirit. I share my experiences, what I wish I would have known, and the steps to consider toward your healing. You are a unique beautifully created child of God knitted together perfectly but living in a world that makes it almost impossible to be healed. Fear not, there is hope here. You are not alone.

A Desperate Journey

Absolutely nothing happens by accident. You hold this book in your hands because you may feel called to fix your reproductive system—the core of your womanhood—which feels very broken, but you don't know where to start. Worse, you might feel alone, like nobody really understands you. Perhaps you have seen many doctors, yet received very few answers. You may be wondering if you will ever feel normal again.

I have been broken in this lifetime. Twice in fact. The second time would be the last time.

I have lived through a desperate and lonely journey. I never realized that I could exhaust my mental and physical wherewithal until I experienced the dramatic changes of perimenopause and, eventually, surgical menopause. I have spent most of my adolescent and adult life fighting my own body and my hormones.

Hormonal changes for me began in junior high school. A friend of mine invited me to join her at a Christian camp the summer after sixth grade. One day in the bathroom at camp, while I was putting on my bathing suit to get ready to swim with the other kids, I stood up in the stall after using the toilet, and I saw streaks of pink blood in the bowl. I cried out to my friend in the next stall, "I think I started my period!" My voice was quivering. She calmly said that I didn't need to worry and that she had tampons with her, but I had heard that tampons could be bad for you, and I felt very scared. She reassured me and reminded me that it would be the only way I could swim. For the next thirty minutes, she coached me under the stall on how to insert the tampon. I felt embarrassed; finally, when it worked, I walked out wondering whether the other kids would notice my awkwardness. I survived the day, all the while feeling peculiar inside like I wanted to cry, and my tummy felt like it was sticking out more than usual. Everything had changed that day, but I couldn't really explain it. Later that evening, sitting around the campfire with my new friends, the camp counselor, who I had developed a crush on, asked if anyone wanted to experience the peace of Christ through accepting Him as their Savior. My heart pounded like a drum in my chest as I walked up to the fire, and I cried like a baby as I said the prayer that would save and protect me for the rest of my life. Two things happened that day. I started my period for the first time, which would begin a life-long struggle with pain and suffering, but I had also met the One who would pull me through it all. I didn't know then how much I would need Him.

Every month after that day was hell. My period never got easier to live with. I thought someday I might outgrow the intensity, but that month never came. I was riddled with extreme premenstrual syndrome (PMS) and heavy bleeding that often lasted for ten days. I had cramps that kept me bedridden and crying fits that kept me hidden under my bed covers. I missed school, felt too bloated to go out, and was unsure if I was even normal. I felt overly emotional, fat, and exhausted and wondered what was wrong with me. I never understood what was taking over every month, but I knew deep inside that something was wrong.

After suffering through many years of heavy periods and monthly bloating, cramping, and PMS, I became pregnant at age twenty-five. Those days of being pregnant with my son were the most wonderful days of my life. I felt such relief. I felt stable for the first time in a decade. What I did not realize then is that my body was stabilized hormonally. Though my hormones were at high levels, as they always are in pregnancy, they were not seesawing before and after my period. I was happy and hormonally harmonized.

But what goes up must come down. I had my son, went back to full-time work after only twelve weeks of maternity leave, and never let up on the gas pedal. Always a driver, always trying to prove myself, I was now juggling motherhood, my career, and trying to be a good wife. My body felt stressed. I got less rest and pushed harder through all the feelings of fatigue, which only increased my imbalance. The years that followed were filled with ups and downs along with high inflammation markers, autoimmune issues, and an addiction to diet pills. I performed well on the outside but was a total wreck on the inside, and nobody knew. I hid the pills in my car in shoe boxes so nobody would know. I had become a wonderful actress. I spent twelve years on those diet pills to keep the facade of energy and stamina going. But I eventually started to truly fall apart. I had to work for two solid years to heal my gut from fungus from the pills, my brain from the toxic load, and my body from the overall exhaustion. Everything had turned upside down including my hormones. After a lot of hard work, I thought I was finally turning a corner, only to draw closer to the age of perimenopause. I started feeling symptoms in my forties, and, as I aged, they grew worse. I struggled through two surgeries for ovarian cysts, cognitive dysfunction, mood changes, and severe anxiety that altered my thinking and my ability to be an executive, mother, wife, and friend.

I now understand that during the perimenopausal transition, many women experience great hormonal and overall bodily system dysregulation. The physical and emotional pain is often so great we can hardly tolerate it, leaving us feeling hopeless. Some fortunate women will have it easy and experience few symptoms. Others will experience them all. Unfortunately, we rarely talk about it. It's a dark secret that few share. Most of us silently suffer as the struggles of depression and anxiety are often only found in the tears that flow down our faces in the shower. We are ashamed to admit that we are changing and cannot control what is happening, and we are terrified. Millions of women are dying inside; some are even being admitted to psychiatric hospitals, medicated for issues of hormonal imbalance. Others are losing their zest for life and no longer find intimacy possible. They feel dry, tired, fat, sweaty, and alone. Twenty-nine million women a year are going through "the change" and have no idea what it means or what is actually happening, and there is very little education, awareness, or support from doctors unless you have thousands of dollars available to pay out of pocket. Having the financial ability to pay for the support needed during perimenopause is out of reach for many women. Even in some of the most modern countries, healthcare for some is still a privilege, not a right. I have personally spent over $40,000 in the last ten years trying to find answers for myself. Doctors often plug holes to solve problems, focusing on treating symptoms rather than underlying causes, but I have been blessed to meet some systems thinkers who look at the body as a whole system and have taught me what that means. They have each played a part in helping me get my life back. But I never would have gotten there if I hadn't become my own advocate for my healing in addition to doctors' care.

My goal—through this book, my "What I Wish I Knew" podcast, and my Meno Coaching (menocoaching.com) practice—is to educate, empower, and give hope to every woman suffering in silence. It's for the woman who quit her job because she needed to find safe spaces for her healing, the woman who is divorced because she felt misunderstood and ashamed of the power of her emotions, and the woman who walks around in a fog wondering why she is so bloated and tired and why she feels as though she is being set on fire at night.

You don't have to pretend anymore. You have what you need to heal: a radical, countercultural love for yourself and the power to embrace your mind, body, and soul. I'm just here to help you tap into them. I pray daily that my resources give you permission and courage enough to speak your truth and to be vulnerable with your pain. Let our voices together be a wakeup call ... the genesis of a revolution! It's our time to heal and find wholeness.

Nothing Starts Without a Trigger

I call my eight years during perimenopause "the Wilderness." My perimenopausal symptoms came in the form of high anxiety, emotional instability, mood swings, and extreme exhaustion. My journey in the Wilderness uncovered more than just hormonal issues; it also revealed my soul's desire to dig deeper into the recesses of the hidden pain of my past.

Trauma has the power to change the brain. It has been scientifically proven that our neurons can reorganize to deal with the pain of the trauma we experience. "As a result of trauma, certain groups of neurons (those related to survival functions) may, over time, connect more strongly with each other while becoming more isolated from the rest of the brain" (Greenberg). Every cell in our body responds to every hard thing we live through. Trauma is something that, unfortunately, my body and brain were very familiar with.

My trauma started early in my life. Following my parents' divorce when I was five years old, I felt lost and abandoned. My father, despite promising to keep his commitment to parenting, went silent for three years after the divorce. When I was eight years old, he decided to reenter my life. But every other Sunday, when he was supposed to visit, he left me waiting at the living room window hoping he would show up. My stomach would fill with knots as I waited, yearning for his embrace. He rarely showed, and I began to inwardly believe I was damaged. My father, unhappy that my mother had moved on, couldn't face picking me up at another man's home. I felt rejected and unlovable at a crucial stage in my life—when I was trying to figure out my place in the world. Even today, I can feel the pit that would open in my stomach as I waited by that window. It was visceral.

Our brains respond to abandonment by creating feelings of insecurity, fear, and shame. By age eight, I had decided that men could not be counted on because they always leave, and that belief hardened like cement in my psyche. Life at home with my mom and stepdad in our new blended family was riddled with stress and anger. My escape was music. I would go into my room and turn up the radio as loud as I could and sing at the top of my lungs to drown out the yelling through the walls. I could *feel* every note. I yearned for dopamine, the pleasure chemical linked to the power of each note. Music brought joy to my soul. It still does to this day. I realize now that I was self-medicating through my ability to *feel* the music. It saved my life many times. I could escape my reality and feel free.

As I managed through my high school and college years, I met a man and fell in love. I remember telling him we needed to get married as soon as possible so I could leave my parents' home to start our own, better, life. Not the best way to begin a marriage. Unfortunately, I couldn't outrun my demons; nor could marriage guarantee healing. My internal dialogue of not being enough and feeling rejected manifested into a need to be perfect. A need to do it all. To be Superwoman. I was convinced that was my purpose. I had an insatiable desire and drive to get to the highest level of achievement at work as well as a heart filled with a desire to be a perfect mom. During this time, God blessed me with my most precious gift in this life—my son. My heart broke open and grew twice its size the day he entered the world, but my perfectionism got the better of me again, and balancing my career and my family sent my life spiraling out of control.

After letting a friend know that I was experiencing major exhaustion from being up all night with my son and trying to launch a career, she suggested a pill that would promise energy and the loss of my baby fat. I was elated. The promise was true; I got skinny and ran around like a rabbit going to work, going to preschool, and cleaning the house. I felt superhuman. But I wasn't. I was actually addicted to diet pills and trying to fill a hole in my heart with incessant work and a desire to achieve professionally. It was never enough. It was a bucket that, no matter how full, felt empty. The truth is, I was empty. I was struggling to feel like my life had any value. The world had promised fulfillment through material things and money, but they failed to satisfy me. I had been convinced that every promotion, every deal I made, every new car would give me the power I sought. Every single day, I told myself that if I just pushed a little harder, if I just kept forging ahead, I would soon arrive wherever I was going.

My extensive travel, insatiable drive, and Type A personality eventually ended my eight-year marriage. I had sworn, watching my parents' divorce, that it would *never* happen to me, but there I was, repeating the cycle. I powered through my divorce, finalizing details, splitting expenses, working twice as hard to keep our house. I don't think I even cried more than once. I was determined to not allow this hardship to impact me or my son. We were moving on. I developed a stronger internal fire to prove myself and show that I was strong. I dated casually and even told my future husband on our first date that I would never remarry. I was Ms. Independent. That same man is now my husband.

After only a year of dating, we fell deeply in love, and I remarried. We had a blended family and worked hard to raise good kids and build a life together. Though we appeared to have the perfect life on the outside, inside I was still striving, working, and relying on the diet pills to keep up with the pace of my life. I was also getting my master's degree. Our kids grew up, and my son was about to graduate from high school. We had finally done it! All my hard work and sacrifices were finally going to pay off. He was going to college, and life for him would be incredible. I was convinced of it. He was kind, loving, and smart. He had the recipe for a successful life. Then, the music stopped.

On Mother's Day, at the age of eighteen, after a lovely family day, my son started bleeding uncontrollably from colitis. The next two years of our lives were a living hell. We spent our days in and out of gastroenterologists' offices and hospitals. At one point, he spent two months in the hospital due to an infection he developed from immunosuppressant drugs. He became so sick from the infection that his organs began to shut down. I still remember sitting in that hospital room while nurses hooked bags of different antibiotics up to his IV and tried every single other therapy they could find to keep him alive. I felt pieces of myself start to die as I watched him withering to skin and bones in front of me. I prayed God would take me instead of him. Something changed in me that day. I was different—a shell, lost and terrified. That day, the Enemy awakened a spirit of fear inside me that I wrestled with throughout my time in the Wilderness. Though I still believed in God, I had moved away from Him to prioritize work and family. Deep inside, as I cried in the hospital, I knew my only hope was Jesus. The One who I had met at Christian camp. The One who promised to never leave or forsake me.

I vividly remember walking down the hallway into the chapel and nearly collapsing as I fell on my knees, begging God for a miracle. My mom was there with me every single day at that hospital, never leaving me emotionally or spiritually. She was, and always has been, my rock. I don't remember much in that chapel except that I was groaning to God because I had no words left. I knew He was hearing a mother's heart for her sweet child. Oh, how Mary must have felt to watch her son suffer on that cross. Nothing is worse in life than watching your child suffer. Nothing.

Then, the most amazing thing happened. We got our miracle. The kind you see in the movies, the kind only God can do. The miracle that shows you that God is big and strong and sovereign. Day by day, the doctors were able to stabilize my son enough for him to have three different surgeries. He had a large part of his colon removed. He had a colostomy bag for two years; then, through an incredible surgery, he was able to have a pouch created in his body that would allow him to lead a normal life again. Not only did he get his life back, but he also developed a passion for helping others and a deep commitment to serving others in healthcare. Today, he is a paramedic and attends nursing school.

But, while I could not thank God enough for this miracle, I also could not let go of the anguish inside. It haunted me. It was only during perimenopause that it dawned on me that I have always lived waiting for the other shoe to drop. As a child, as an adult, and especially through my later menopause transition, it has been with me like an unwanted spirit. I never truly felt safe in my body or in my life. And a body that never feels safe is always trying to survive. It's always in fight or flight, always prioritizing surviving over thriving. I had never experienced thriving. I needed to be prepared to defend myself at all times just in case things got out of control. This realization came to me in the Wilderness, like a light coming on in a dark room, but it didn't make life any easier. I developed deep-rooted fears: fear about my son getting sick again, fear that he might die, and, worse, fear that it was my fault. It was my work schedule, my divorce, my pressure on him to do well in school. I was the reason that he almost died. These thoughts played over in my head like the music of my teen years, but instead of increasing my joy, they brought me to tears. This constant rumination and the stress of trying to hold my whole universe together set off a series of events inside and outside of me that triggered my entrance into the Wilderness.

What I Wish I Knew About the Enemy

We have an Enemy; his name is Satan. He has the ability to steal, kill, and destroy; to allow things into our lives that open doors for us to condemn ourselves. For years, I was so driven and so determined not to fail that I never questioned myself. I was confident that I was able to survive it all. I was proud of my fierce strength; in fact, I wore it like a badge of honor. What is clear to me now is that as we age, and as the body goes through this dramatic period of change, we feel less and less like the person we once knew physically and even mentally. We interpret this lack of energy as weakness, but, in reality, our bodies are trying to conserve energy. It's the body's natural way of protecting itself, of trying to keep us alive, of trying to make every molecule of energy available for this massive transition. But we override this natural function, we don't pause to reflect and review where we can implement change, we keep going as if nothing is happening. All the while, society reinforces that we should live in a continuous loop of focused ambition for more money and a size four body, while appearing as if nothing at all is wrong. We push through and dig deep and motivate ourselves with bumper stickers and Instagram feeds, certain that we can fix the problem if we *just try harder*. Permimenopause was begging me to shift gears, to slow down, to find myself again. I resisted it with force. I was afraid of stopping, of facing myself. I was afraid of what I would find or who I would be in the stillness.

But the body keeps score. If we don't listen to the inner need to downshift, we pay a price. I was unwilling to face the fact that my body, my energy levels, and even my brain were changing. It was too much for me. Consequently, the Enemy saw an open door and walked in, bringing with him the spirit of fear and anxiety that took over my life as my adrenaline hit record highs. By not dealing with my past, I entered a war, a spiritual war with my Enemy within my soul. This battle has been at the center of my journey. The good news is that God never left my side; I was never alone in the Wilderness. He brought my inner brokenness to the surface, one memory at a time, for my healing and for His glory, but I had to fight for every single piece of ground.

Jesus in the Wilderness

Entering the Wilderness of perimenopause is no joke, yet we joke about it all the time. Our society makes fun of something debilitating, which breaks my heart. *Menopause the Musical* is a parody on women being forgetful, sexually dysfunctional, and soaked in night sweat. It brought in millions of dollars and still sells out in days. I remember going to see it with my mom in my early forties wondering if it was, in fact, funny to experience these things. I truly believe that this attempt to downplay this change is why we feel the need to remain silent as women. This kind of attention gives society permission to laugh at something extremely serious and even life threatening. There is nothing humorous about the Wilderness. It is fiercely dark, and, some days, it's all we can do to just put one foot in front of the other, sometimes one hour at a time. The anxiety, night sweats, insomnia, brain fog, and extreme fatigue are beyond anything one would laugh about.

In the New Testament of the Bible, "wilderness" is translated from the Greek word "eremos," which means an isolated place.

"Wilderness" is also defined in the dictionary as an "uninhabited or uncultivated area." The Wilderness of perimenopause is somewhere we have never been before; there are no rules, no instructions on how to navigate. It's a feeling of being lost, alone, forgotten, and far from home. I believe that this is God's purpose for this period in our lives. It's not that He wants us to suffer, but, rather, that our time in the Wilderness will serve a purpose if we are willing to explore the terrain. The menopausal transition for many is about being pushed far enough to find ourselves again, but it can feel very lonely. My only comfort was in knowing others had gone through long periods in the wilderness and survived. Even Jesus.

Many biblical characters spent time in the wilderness. Moses and the Israelites, Job, John the Baptist, and Jesus Himself. In Matthew 3:16, we find Jesus being baptized by John the Baptist and the Spirit of God filling him. The Spirit cried, "This is my Son, whom I love; with him I am well pleased." Yet, in Matthew 4:1, "Jesus was led by the Spirit into the wilderness to be tempted by the devil." He fasted for forty days and nights; it was at his lowest point that he was tempted and underwent trial and pain. The Israelites spent forty years in the wilderness while God led them the long way to the Red Sea. What should have been an eleven-day journey took forty years as God used this period to strengthen their faith and to teach them to lean on Him. He showed Himself to them daily with just enough light and grace to get them to the Promised Land after forty years.

So, what does this all mean? It means that the Wilderness is *allowed* by God. He is sovereign, which means that nothing happens in our lives without His consent. I have held onto this belief for the entirety of this wild ride. There is a purpose in the pain to grow into deeper levels of ourselves than we ever thought possible. But that is of little comfort during the darkest hours when we can't see the way out, when we are crying out for relief, and when we fear we won't make it one more day. The purpose is hidden in the muck and mire of trying to pull ourselves out of the darkness. But sometimes we need to touch the darkness so we are able to recognize the light.

The Valley of OCD

After my son's illness, as my constant battle with anxiety and ruminations hit an all-time high, I was diagnosed with obsessive-compulsive disorder (OCD). We make light of it today, describing it as people who are overly clean or obsessed with alphabetizing their food labels and drawers, but it's so much more serious than people realize. OCD comes in many different forms, and our society is severely undereducated regarding how this imbalance in neurotransmitters impacts people's daily lives. Some find it hard to leave their homes for fear of germs; some wash the skin off their hands trying to compulsively clean; and others cannot stop their minds from ruminating.

My OCD manifested for the first time when I was only ten years old as my transition into puberty began. This was my first indication, a foreshadowing, that my OCD was hormone related. Once I began having periods, I would cry to my mother each month right before they would start and tell her that I was scared because I kept having bad thoughts. She would soothe me and say, "Just think good thoughts and push the bad ones away, and it will be okay." For a long time, it worked. I was able to control the power the thoughts had over my life by pushing them out of my mind and replacing them with thoughts that made me happy.

I also obsessed over the weight gain caused by my periods. I weighed myself daily, measuring my success and happiness through the number on the scale. I restricted myself to carrots and grapes for days. I did not realize it at the time, but control was what I was looking for; and control, or a lack of control, is at the center of OCD. This obsession for control continued in my life, manifesting as diet pill use and perfectionism, and would come with a vengeance during my menopause transition. As with most things, I would realize through the journey that there were several roots to the tree of OCD, and my body was responding to each and every experience, trauma, and cry for freedom.

I remember during puberty listening to music or watching television and having the ability to experience the music or a television show as if I had composed it or written it. I could feel things with an incredible visceral intensity. I struggled to understand why these intense emotions would come over me. Now I know that I am an empath. "Empaths have an extremely reactive neurological system. We don't have the same filters that other people do to block out stimulation. As a consequence, we absorb into our own bodies both positive and stressful energies around us" (Orloff 2).

Empaths are feeling-oriented people that are wired genetically to have a highly-sensitive connection to emotion and to people and their feelings. It is my greatest blessing and biggest curse. While I can command a room with my energy, I can also crash from the weight of a tense discussion full of great emotion. This predisposition complicated my struggle as I felt everything physically and mentally in extremes.

What I Wish I Knew About Trauma

As I researched my diagnosis, I learned that OCD is an over-focus chemical issue. "Compared to the brains of normal controls, the brains of our OCD volunteers showed hypermetabolic activity in the orbital frontal cortex" (Schwartz and Begley 62). This hyperfocus served me well in my early days of striving to achieve at all costs, but it had turned on me. During my time in the Wilderness, that same intense focus became torture as the ruminations came in the form of intrusive thoughts that I could not control. "Obsessive-compulsive disorder is a neuropsychiatric disease marked by distressing, intrusive, unwanted thoughts (the obsession part) that trigger intense urges to perform ritualistic behaviors (the compulsion part)" (Schwartz and Begley 52). When I met with an OCD psychologist, I learned that people who suffer from OCD are often CEOs, doctors, and very successful executives. They are people who persevere and focus on their goals no matter the cost. This has been my whole post-adolescent life. I learned that OCD is a communication error in the brain where the message gets stuck, and it feels like you can't put the brakes on your looping thoughts. It has to do with too much glutamate and not enough GABA (both small-molecule neurotransmitters) in the brain, as well as a problem with serotonin synthesis in the brain. OCD causes moments of heightened focus as the glutamate excites the brain and causes ruminating thoughts. However, the OCD psychologist told me several times that it was not curable or treatable. I found myself going from being depressed at this news to outraged. How could a therapist play God? Why would they train my brain to believe this? How was this helpful? I decided I would never go back and would defy the label. I was determined to get to the root of my suffering.

Afterall, I hadn't always been that way. I went back into the research, looking for the "why." What I found was both liberating and complex. As I scoured research articles in psychiatry, I found that

OCD is often triggered by childhood trauma. It is also triggered by inflammation in the body and brain. This information was eye opening as I began to see that my situation was multifaceted. "For a small percentage of obsessive-compulsive disorder cases exhibiting additional neuropsychiatric symptoms, it was proposed that neuroinflammation occurs in the basal ganglia as an auto-immune response to infections. However, it is possible that elevated neuroinflammation, inducible by a diverse range of mechanisms, is important throughout the cortico-striato-thalamo-cortical circuit of OCD" (Attwells et al. Abstract). All of this was starting to make some sense. I had been "diagnosed" with autoimmune disease years before, and I had experienced trauma. Had the switches been turned on without my permission? I suddenly found myself facing the trauma of my early years, the pain of my son's illness, my OCD label, and the Wilderness all at once. It was the perfect storm.

The interesting part about genes, hormones, and trauma is that we don't know where one starts and another one stops. They are a dance. They are interchangeable, and they impact each other to create a fabric of who we become, how we interpret the world, and, most importantly, how we respond. "Yes, our biology can affect our mental state. However, humans' multifaceted experiences cannot be understood as isolated events. They're intrinsically connected to the whole life history and experiences of the individual" (Leaf 39). I wish I knew earlier in my life how many pieces there were to my puzzle, how both the trauma in life and my biology had contributed to my imbalances. God designed us for harmony, but we often don't get to the root of our personal or biological challenges until we are very sick or overwhelmed by the transition into menopause. The body knows exactly what it needs, but we often ignore the whispers until it is screaming.

Menstrual Conditions That Plague: PMDD, PCOS, Endometriosis, and Adenomyosis

No discussion of menstrual issues would be complete without some explanation of the complex conditions that some women unfortunately experience. Many women suffer with one or multiple conditions (comorbidity) for many years before entering perimenopause, while others find they arise or become worse during the transition into perimenopause as the body becomes more and more hormonally unstable. Because our Western medical culture tends to focus on treating symptoms and often lacks an integrated approach, treating any of these conditions can be very difficult as they are complex and multifaceted. The comorbidity yet often separate treatment of these conditions is a prime example that our entire system of women's health is on fire with no systems thinkers to heal it (or them).

Premenstrual Dysphoric Disorder/PMDD

PMDD is basically PMS on steroids. It impacts women mentally, physically, and emotionally. It can cause moodiness, extreme food cravings, bloating, and anxiety. PMDD impacts women two to three weeks out of the month, and, thus, can be debilitating. I was diagnosed with PMDD and told I was emotionally sensitive, hormonal, and basically mental. The diagnosis nearly crushed me and left me feeling hopeless, which only magnified my emotional response. What I wish I knew then that I know now is that PMDD is actually a sensitivity to the changing hormone levels a woman experiences each month. "PMDD is often thought of as an abnormal response to normal hormonal changes. Traditional lab testing often indicates that their hormone levels are 'normal' furthering the frustration and dismissal of their concerns" (Brighten). PMDD requires an approach that looks at all aspects of a woman's history including past trauma. I was that woman. In fact, it has been proven that women who have experienced trauma early in life are more likely to suffer from PMDD. In a study in Australia, eighty-three percent of women with PMDD had experienced early life trauma (Kulkarni et al.). Treating this condition is a combination of gut healing, estrogen balancing, thyroid support, supplementation, and often therapy. It's complex and requires a multifaceted approach, but it is possible to heal from PMDD.

Polycystic Ovary Syndrome/PCOS

PCOS is a common menstrual condition that affects five to ten percent of women in their childbearing years. Women with this condition produce abnormal amounts of androgen hormone and often develop small cysts along the outer edge of their ovaries. PCOS can cause extreme weight gain, excessive body hair growth, elongated menstrual cycles or missed periods, depression, and exhaustion. The exact cause of PCOS is unknown, but there is some evidence that it might be an endocrine issue, particularly an issue with the hypothalamus. "[A] growing body of evidence supports the notion that the pathogenesis underlying PCOS may lie upstream in the central nervous system regulation of the ovaries, especially the abnormal activation of the hypothalamic gonadotropin-releasing hormone (GnRH) neurons" (Gaspar). If there was ever a complex set of challenges, PCOS is it. The approach to healing PCOS, too, is multifaceted. In my practice, Meno Coaching, we've seen several patients with PCOS who previously had been treated with multiple antidepressants, birth control, and even Metformin (a diabetes medication). They are worse, not better. Our approach includes hormone balancing, reducing inflammation, and supporting metabolism, gut health, and blood sugar through sound nutrition. We also focus on healing the mind through prayer, meditation, and breathing techniques. As you can imagine, PCOS is not an easy fix; it takes commitment and experienced practitioners.

Endometriosis and Adenomyosis

Both endometriosis and adenomyosis are conditions where endometrial tissue—which lines the uterus—grows where it shouldn't. With endometriosis, the tissue grows outside the uterus, often on the ovaries and fallopian tubes and/or within the pelvic cavity. With adenomyosis, the tissue grows within the uterine muscle, deep within the uterine wall and can cause the abdomen to protrude. Both conditions can cause heavy bleeding, pelvic pain, and infertility. And both have been proven to be influenced by genetic factors. After genetic testing, I found that I had an affinity for adenomyosis, which was further complicated by having my cysts removed. It is also clear that both of these conditions appear to subside after menopause. This is no surprise as estrogen decreases significantly then, thus limiting its power to grow the endometrial cells and tissue.

I share this information because these conditions are often windows of insight into what women may experience later as they enter into perimenopause and menopause. Awareness and being proactive leads to earlier and more effective management at all stages.

The Deep Wilderness of Perimenopause

"Perimenopause is when your body starts transitioning to menopause. During this transition, your ovaries begin producing less hormones, causing your menstrual cycle to become erratic or irregular. At this time your body is moving toward the end of your reproductive years ... Other physical changes and symptoms can occur as your body adjusts to different hormone levels. Perimenopause begins about eight to ten years before menopause" (Cleveland Clinic). Yes, eight to ten years of ups and downs, and yet women are abandoned in the Wilderness with limited guidance and support.

The most terrifying aspect of perimenopause is dealing with the unknown—the unknown about how we will feel from day to day, the uncontrollable emotions, and the shame-filled body changes. It is so turbulent that we can only see what is directly in front of us, but we must still run the race of life full throttle. What I quickly realized was that not only did I not know how to navigate it all, I also felt like there was nothing holding me together. I felt completely out of control. "Perimenopause is the transitional stage into menopause during which the ovaries start to run out of good eggs. In reaction, the brain starts sending either stronger or erratic amounts of FSH [follicle-stimulating hormone] to the ovaries, thus yielding more eggs than usual and promoting pregnancy. This also results in increased and often fluctuating estrogen levels. At times, ovulation does not happen at all" (Hawkins 54). Those strong erratic signals were at the root of my emotional roller coaster. There is truly a wild ride going on in our bodies, and, being an empath, I felt it all. I also felt that God had gone quiet in my life. I could no longer feel Him or hear His voice, the voice that had once been so familiar, so comforting. I felt totally alone. I started to wonder if the God I had so faithfully believed in was no longer hearing my prayers. I started to doubt my faith for the first time in my life. I started to believe the lie that I was paying for every bad thing I had ever done in my life. I started to believe that the other shoe had finally dropped, just like I had always thought it would.

My first step into the Wilderness was full of fear, and my symptoms were very consistent. I had constant anxiety that would ebb and flow with my menstrual cycle, which had become totally erratic and was longer and heavier than ever before. I felt what can only be described as a major tremor in the inner core of my body but for no reason. I felt like a balloon as I was constantly bloated, and my stomach ached. My pants were tight, my skin was stretched, and I felt like I was living in someone else's body. I started to have days of extreme exhaustion and crying fits mid-cycle and then again just before my cycle began. I had periods of brain fog and disconnection that made me feel like I was not really "here." I even started getting two cycles a month. At that point, I had my hormone levels tested. My progesterone levels were very low, and my estrogen levels were very high. I was told that it was the ratio of progesterone to estrogen that mattered, and mine was drastically imbalanced. I was "estrogen dominant." So I was prescribed progesterone to help balance my system. While progesterone therapy helped manage my sleep and some of the anxiety, I still could not control my overall feeling of being "off."

My eating habits had also changed dramatically. I knew I was going to start my cycle because I would inhale a bag of Oreos at night and then still run out to grab ice cream. I had no control over my eating, which made me gain weight and made me feel worse after I came down from the sugar high. I felt ashamed and powerless. Eating would temporarily take these feelings away, but the feel-good chemicals would inevitably run out, and I would be left with only myself and the empty packets scattered around me. I was self-medicating and didn't know it. The Enemy knew my weakness and where to attack. My body was crying out for harmony, but I was ill-informed about all the broken pieces in my mind and body that needed healing. Perimenopause is a system in constant flux. And I hate change. Everything felt so uncertain, even my physical state, and I yearned for stability. I felt this uncomfortable, yet strange, connection to my body. I could feel the fact that it was my hormones causing my emotional turmoil, my mood swings, my anxiety. I *knew* my body was connected but could not find a way to stop the turbulence. The unpredictable perimenopause journey is an ebb and flow of the body trying to find homeostasis, but it was causing my life to become unmanageable. Being estrogen dominant was always my problem. It was why I always felt so bloated and why my cravings were so high. My estrogen levels were at 600 to 700 pg/mL (picograms per milliliter), two to three times what they should have been, which not only caused immediate discomfort but also created a perfect environment for cancer. "Previous studies have shown that women with high blood levels of estradiol have an increased risk of breast cancer both before and after menopause. Ovarian cancer is the most fatal of the gynecological cancers worldwide, with no screening test and therefore typically late-stage diagnosis" (Johansson et al. 1). I was privileged enough to have the best doctors money could buy. Not everyone does. We tried progesterone, we tried diets, we tried gut healing. We tried everything. I still could not get my estrogen under control. I increased the progesterone again and tried some estrogen metabolizers, which brought some relief and a small glimmer of hope.

I started to feel better as I slowly experienced some healing, and my hormones balanced a bit. But then, out of nowhere, my estrogen soared, and I climbed right back onto the roller coaster. My schedule was hectic, and I was traveling a lot for work. The stress and the pressure of being a senior partner at a global firm was getting to me. At the height of my perimenopausal nightmare, I was by myself in a hotel in Canada full of fear. I was supposed to start my period any day. I was shaking with anxiety while my brain ran a million miles an hour. I felt overwhelming fear for absolutely no reason. I was cramping and starving, and my breasts were aching. I ordered room service and inhaled a stack of fries and a cheeseburger, and then ordered two desserts. My hunger was insatiable. I could not control my appetite, and I felt like a stranger in my own body. It was one of the worst days of my life, and I wanted so badly to be in my home, under the duvet covers, waiting for my cycle to pass. I was terrified of being alone in my hotel room and even more terrified of going to my client the next day, afraid that they would notice that I was spiraling out of control. All of this just because I was supposed to start my period!

So I did what I always do, I searched for a sense of control, but this time it would change my outlook and shift my perspective entirely as it led me to explore the world of holistic medicine.

As I sat in the bed in my lonely hotel room unable to sleep, I started researching doctors, counselors, and anyone who knew anything about anxiety and PMS. I stumbled upon a woman who specialized in hair analysis of people with hormonal dysregulation. And—the God part of it all—she lived in Canada. Moreover, she answered my email at 9:00 pm that night and took my call thirty minutes later. It was surreal. She was incredible: caring, loving, and a Christian. I will never forget her or that moment. She said she had worked with many women with similar issues, and she could help me. She mentioned pyrrole disorder (also called Pyroluria); I had never heard of it before. She explained that it was an overproduction of the enzyme pyrrole in urine, which absorbs zinc and vitamin B6 and expels them via urination and, thus, deprives the body of them. Zinc and vitamin B6 are crucial for calming the nervous system and increasing GABA, the calming neurotransmitter. I was overwhelmed but hopeful for the first time in a long time. I got off the phone with her, ordered a hair analysis test, and started my research.

What I Wish I Knew About the Brain and Pyrrole Disorder

I read for hours on everything I could find related to nutrients, pyrrole disorder, and the endocrine system. An overabundance of pyrroles causes a depletion of zinc and vitamin B6. This lack of zinc and vitamin B6, in turn, causes anxiety, depression, PMS, and even ADHD (attention-deficit/hyperactivity disorder). Many people are given antidepressant medications to treat the *symptoms*, which can actually worsen pyrrole disorder because the antidepressants themselves have been shown to also deplete zinc and vitamin B6.

That night in Canada was a pivotal moment for me. It was the night I decided to become my own advocate, my own physician. It was my first step into learning how to understand my deficiencies and how to heal myself.

Some Answers

My hair analysis results came back three weeks later. Sure enough, I had pyrrole disorder. I also had other major nutrient deficiencies that suggested high levels of stress in my system. It sounded scary, but, in many ways, I felt relief. I finally had some answers. My symptoms weren't my fault; I wasn't a failure; I wasn't suffering because I wasn't strong enough or because I hadn't tried hard enough. I just needed to get my system back into balance. I started taking vitamin B6 P5P and zinc picolinate twice a day, and, within only thirty days, I noticed my PMS had improved by fifty percent. I felt better and had more clarity; I felt calmer and more in control. But I was not healed.

Month after month, I unpeeled another layer of the onion. I went to Mensah Medical, a specialty clinic for biochemical imbalances, after reading Dr. William Walsh's research on pyrrole disorder. I worked with their best doctors in the field of anxiety and PMS and learned that I also had the MTHFR gene mutation. People who have this gene mutation are unable to metabolize folate, which not only helps cleanse excess estrogen out of the body but also promotes neurotransmitter synthesis in the brain. Without enough folate, we can't properly metabolize or produce enough serotonin, dopamine, epinephrine, or adrenaline during the methylation cycle (a biochemical reaction inherent in human metabolism) to be happy, calm, and balanced. A lack of folate thus causes undermethylation, a condition with symptoms that include anxiety, joint pain, competitive personality traits, perfectionism, high achievement, and OCD ... yes, OCD!! In addition to taking zinc and vitamin B6, I started a special kind of folate supplement called L-methylfolate. Immediately, I felt calm and totally normalized as if it was the missing puzzle piece.

But then, after one week of treatment, the anxiety got worse. I called the doctor and was told that my undermethylation had quickly turned to overmethylation and that I should pull back on the dosage. My journey was getting more and more complex. So, once again, I researched. I read every blog written by experts on MTHFR and landed on that of Dr. Ben Lynch, the authority on MTHFR and its effects on the methylation cycle. I read his book *Dirty Genes* and studied his podcasts regarding the importance of methylation on numerous physiological processes. "Think of those two hundred functions as gardens located throughout our body. Just as gardens need water, so do those processes need methyl groups. The methylation cycle is like an irrigation system that draws water from a clean lake and distributes it to all the gardens. If something blocks or disrupts the irrigation system, some or all of those two hundred gardens won't get the water they need" (RN Labs quoting Dr. Ben Lynch). These processes include not only neurotransmitter synthesis, but hormone metabolism, detoxification, mood regulation, and even weight management. He explained that too much of a good thing is a bad thing. The graphics in *Dirty Genes* showed the pathways of folate and illustrated how some people need folinic acid (another type of folate) and vitamin B12 in small amounts to go downstream to turn into folate to help the brain. I ordered folinic acid with B12 from his site and started to test it on myself. It worked. I started to feel better. Dr. Lynch also emphasized that pushing folate without cleaning up the oxidative stress in the body can wreak havoc. Glutathione, an antioxidant, helps this process. Dr. Lynch taught me two things: first, the body was a system, and, second, I had to heal my body through my own education and internal wisdom. I had two gifts from God: I was gritty and resilient at my very core, and I was more curious and determined to find answers than even I knew. Little did I know just how much I would need these strengths as I continued to walk through the Wilderness.

Estrogen Likes to Grow Things

I was armed with information and power. I came to believe I would finally get better and healthier, but then I started to battle with regular ovarian cysts. Since the MTHFR gene mutation makes it hard to clear out the bad estrogen, I decided to get off the birth control pill. I had been on it for more than twenty years. Often when a woman gets off birth control pills, her body has a difficult time coming back to its natural baseline. It's almost as if it has forgotten how to function normally, and all of those suppressed hormones come back with a vengeance.

I found a doctor of osteopathic medicine (DO) who looked beyond the obvious acute symptoms to causality and determined that my estrogen dominance was causing my cysts. She treated me with increased natural progesterone to balance my high estrogen levels. Estrogen lines the uterus and increases cell production. It grows the endometrium (the lining of the uterus), but, when out of control, it can cause endometriosis for some women and even grow ovarian endometriomas. When estrogen is balanced with progesterone, our bodies feel "happy." Progesterone had helped, but, eventually, the cysts took over. It is important to note that women experience functional cysts every month when they ovulate; these are follicles that hold and then release an egg each cycle. Functional cysts, however, don't get very big, and they naturally break down after ovulation. They should never get to the size where one cannot button their pants or comfortably sit down.

My cysts were so big that I looked like I was three months pregnant; I stared at myself in the mirror with sadness and disgust. My body continued to turn on me no matter what I did. I felt powerless again. I would wake up during the night and sob in the bathroom as the pressure of another large cyst felt like a knife stabbing my stomach. I was anxious, a ball of nerves. I contacted my doctor and was rushed into a vaginal scan. My cyst was over four centimeters and was pushing on my bladder. My doctor suggested surgery as she was sure the cyst would continue to grow and eventually burst, which would cause immense pain. My estrogen levels were through the roof. She explained that as cysts grow, they make their own estrogen, which exacerbates already high estrogen levels. I had no choice. In the summer of 2017, I had my first ovarian cyst surgically removed. The surgeon reported that the surgery was complex and that he was almost unable to take the cyst out without removing my ovary because of how enmeshed it was with my tissue. I was so grateful because one of my biggest fears in life was having my ovaries removed. Go figure!

While cyst removal is very common and not even very painful, it turns hormones upside down. Because my cyst was already dysregulating my system by making its own hormones, taking it out caused both my estrogen and progesterone levels to quickly drop. I remember thinking, "What goes up must come down." I remember being on the couch in tears, trembling with anxiety and waves of depression. I had never experienced depression before, and I became worried that it would never lift. I was sore, tired, and completely defeated. My mom prayed over me, and all I could do was listen to worship music and pray. My doctor increased my supplements; finally, after three weeks, things calmed down, and I started to feel much better. I thought that maybe it was all over. I thought that perhaps I was finally getting my miracle! I was wrong.

What I Wish I Knew About Birth Control and PMS

I wish I had known a long time ago that birth control pills dysregulate the entire natural function of a woman's body. I started the pill at the early age of sixteen, but I never felt right on it. I would always cry before my period. I was heavy, bloated, and my breasts would get so big I could hardly close my bra. Birth control pills are prescribed like candy for PMS, acne, painful periods, heavy periods, cysts, and endometriosis. It's a doctor's go-to medication for many female issues. Here is the truth. "Rather than containing natural hormones, they're synthetic versions of endogenous estradiol and progesterone, and Mother Nature has never seen these at any time in human evolution. In a sense, these synthetic hormones are endocrine disruptors—chemicals that can be thought of as pseudo-hormones … If you went to the toxicology site at the US National Institutes of Health, you would find the ingredients of birth control pills listed as endocrine disruptors" (Gersh).

For these reasons, I will always believe that my hormonal problems started much earlier than I realized due to synthetic hormones floating around in my body for over nineteen years. I wish I would have realized that PMS was a cry from my body for natural hormonal balance. Instead, I was told by several doctors that I was just unlucky and needed birth control or antidepressants. I may have had a few minor feelings of depression during this whole experience, but that is not surprising considering what I was going through. But I was *not* depressed when those doctors told me I was! I was hormonally dysregulated. But how much easier was it to give me a pill to serve as a band-aid for my issues instead of looking for the cause?

Nobody had the inclination to suggest deeper investigation. I wish I had known that there was more to the puzzle—gut issues, genetic issues, nutrient issues, stress management issues, adrenal issues, and many more. I finally just accepted that PMS would be with me until the day my periods ended, which would have to be okay with me. At least I knew it would one day come to an end. But I was young, and I had no idea that this was only an early indicator of what was to come.

What I Wish I Knew About the Gut and the Estrobolome

What continued for me was a series of ovarian cysts. They would come and go. Sometimes I would be able to get rid of them, other times I couldn't. At my doctor's suggestion, I tried everything from diindolylmethane (DIM) to calcium D-glucarate, supplements that are known to help metabolize and clear out excess bad estrogen. I became a student of holistic medicine. I met with functional doctors and nutritionists, but my most important realization was that I had to learn what my body needed and educate myself on what my symptoms were telling me. Symptoms, I learned, are information. And I needed data.

I received a lot of information from Michael Smith, a naturopathic doctor (ND) and the founder of Planet Naturopath. Michael specializes in testing for underlying causes of health challenges. When we met, I learned more in thirty minutes than I had in months. I realized through my experience with Michael that although other doctors had tried different therapies, they never explained how they interacted with my body. He taught me about the power of getting my gut healed. Other doctors had suggested the usual protocols for this, but nobody did testing ... not one test! So no one had delved into the science behind my issues. Michael was different; he was a systems thinker. He had me take the GI-MAP™ (GI Microbial Assay

Plus) test, and the pieces of the puzzle came together. I learned that I had gut dysbiosis (disruption of gut bacterial homeostasis) and yeast in my gut and blood stream. I also had bad gut bacteria and, at one point, H. pylori. I began to treat my imbalances with probiotics. I also learned how gut health impacted brain health. Years of dieting had led me to bad food habits and malnutrition, which prevented my body from making neurotransmitters critical for balancing my mood and hormones. I had been conditioned by a diet culture to believe that a skinny body was a healthy body. My body was under constant stress from lack of real nutrition, which contributed to my high cortisol and fight or flight response. We need food for fuel and enough healthy fat to make hormones! I was afraid of fat! I learned that eating enough, eating well, and taking care of my body had to be a priority if I was going to get better. So, I started eating a good breakfast with gluten-free bread and almond butter with a half of a banana, followed by a midmorning snack, and lunch at noon that included protein and a vegetable. I always eat dinner by 6:00 pm and include more protein and brown rice or potatoes with a vegetable. Eating this way served my body and gave me the ability to feel calm while managing my blood sugar, which is important for cortisol regulation. But even with all of this new knowledge, I still had an issue with my estrogen.

I mentioned estrogen dominance earlier—the imbalance in the ratio between estrogen and progesterone. It doesn't always occur due to high levels of estrogen itself. Sometimes we actually have the right amount of estrogen, but the progesterone can be so low that we experience estrogen-dominance symptoms. This is particularly true during perimenopause when the ovaries begin to shut down, which depletes progesterone in the body. Additionally, sometimes estrogen dominance occurs when women struggle to clear out estrogen from their bodies due to genetic mutations and *overall gut health*. "The human gut microbiome exerts both local and wide-reaching effects. For example, a subset of microbes within the gastrointestinal tract impacts the metabolism of the various forms of estrogens and the balance of circulating and excreted hormone levels. These microbes are collectively referred to as the estrobolome. Microbes in the estrobolome produce beta-glucuronidase. This enzyme alters estrogens into their active forms, which can bind to estrogen receptors and influence estrogen-dependent physiological processes. In general, the more beta-glucuronidase that the microbes in your gut produce, the less estrogen is excreted out of the body so that more remains within the body to be recirculated, bind to receptors and exert their influence on various physiologic processes" (Weinberg). Estrogen that is recirculated within the body can cause a myriad of health problems. If met with a genetic predisposition to cancer, it can be deadly.

Estrogen makes things grow—the lining of the uterus, cells, cysts, fibroids, and sometimes cancer. Progesterone balances estrogen and keeps the uterine lining from building up these cells, but it can only do so much when a woman is trying to combat a dysregulated system, recirculated estrogen, and genetic mutations. An imbalance favoring estrogen made me focused and energized. Because of its impact on serotonin and dopamine, the estrogen imbalance made me assertive and helped me be the driver of my life. "Estrogens affect a wide array of cognitive processes by altering transmission in various neurotransmitter systems. There is growing evidence that estrogens affect dopamine-dependent cognitive processes" (Almey et al. Part 3). In many ways, I think I loved my estrogen dominance, until I hated it. Despite having my ovarian cyst removed and starting on gut healing therapies, my estrogen was not cooperating.

Navigating the Hell of Healthcare

In the summer of 2018, desperate for healing, I visited an OB-GYN at my mom's suggestion. She had seen this OB-GYN and convinced me it was a good idea to get another opinion. As I drove to the appointment, I cried and prayed for answers once again. I walked in feeling a mix of hopelessness and exhaustion. I was met with zero grace for my situation. The doctor said my hormones were normal and that I was going through perimenopause, which causes fluctuations in hormones. She diagnosed me with PMDD, which, at the time, I knew nothing about, and she never explained it. She also said I was depressed and needed Prozac. When I tried to explain that I wasn't depressed but tired and emotional, she discounted me and sent me on my way. I cried all the way home wondering if anyone cared about the struggles I was facing. I knew deep inside my issues were hormonal.

Once again, I went back to the drawing board. This time, I found the North American Menopause Society (NAMS) website. I scrolled through their list of menopause practitioners until I found a woman who I will call Dr. M. She had kind and caring eyes, and her background was treating women entering menopause. She was a certified national expert! Like a relentless dog with a bone, I scheduled an appointment for June 2019.

Dr. M.'s office overlooked the ocean. Just walking in, I felt peaceful. Her office was quiet, and the office staff was incredible. I walked in and opened my mouth for a sentence, which instantly turned into sobbing. She listened and handed me a tissue. It was like a breath of fresh air and peace to my soul. I couldn't believe it, she got it. We talked for an hour. She made some adjustments to my hormones, and she promised she would keep working with me until we found balance. Little did I know how much she would impact my life.

Dr. M. and I worked on testing and balancing my hormone levels every month, but, once again, my estrogen was out of control. Dr. M. is the most loving, kind, and compassionate menopause specialist I have ever known. Not only did she work with my hormones, but she was open and even eager to leverage my work with functional doctors as we partnered on my healing journey. Her dedication has been nothing short of angelic. She listened, supported me, called on the weekends, and fought for me every step of the way. For the first time since entering the Wilderness, I finally felt like I was understood. Unfortunately, the roller coaster continued.

Later in 2020, the familiar ovarian pain came back, but this time it was worse. I was unable to walk from the pain and unable to eat. I had another large ovarian cyst; I couldn't even button my pants because my belly stuck out like that of a pregnant woman again. After a full year of treatment, Dr. M. recommended that I meet with a surgeon, who suggested a second surgery for cyst removal. The surgery went much smoother this time; however, my hormones lagged, and it took longer than expected for them to come back. But as always, when they did, I was full of estrogen. I managed through each day after surgery with all the tools in my toolbox, from supplements to acupuncture to relaxation techniques. I went down to working four days per week to lessen my workload. I walked daily, I prayed, and I asked God to heal me. I was managing.

Genes Tell a Story

As I continued to work on my health, Michael Smith and I continued to search for deeper answers to my challenges. I asked if I should consider genetic testing. I had read about it during my MTHFR research as a way to gain insight into the body's genetic predispositions that impact hormones. I climbed back into research and learned about gene expression, a fascinating area of science. I learned that we all have what are termed genetic SNPs (single nucleotide polymorphisms), which are genetic variations that each of us has in our bodies, our own unique DNA. SNPs can help us identify areas of our genetic code associated with disease or predisposition. I decided to get tested. I literally held my breath as we got on the call to discuss my results. I was absolutely sure there was something there for me; I knew it in my gut and in my heart. I was right, so right. It was there. I had eight out of ten gene mutations for an ESR1 gene SNP. ESR1 is an estrogen-sensitive gene that can cause breast and ovarian cancer. "Ovarian cancer remains the leading cause of death due to gynecologic malignancy. Estrogen-related pathways genes, such as estrogen receptors (ESR1 and ESR2) and their coregulators, proline-, glutamic acid-, and leucine-rich protein 1 (PELP), and proto-oncogene tyrosine protein kinase c-Src (SRC) are involved in ovarian cancer induction and development ..." (Englert-Golan et al. Abstract).

We also found that I had a mutation in my COMT gene, which affects dopamine, serotonin, and estrogen levels. According to Dr. Ben Lynch, a mutated COMT gene is either too "slow" or too "fast." In *Dirty Genes*, Dr. Lynch describes a woman he treated with a slow COMT: "Margo's slow COMT was slow to clear catechols, estrogen, dopamine, norepinephrine, and epinephrine from her system. As a result, her levels of these compounds tended to be high. The extra estrogen gave Margo glowing skin and good sexual function, but it also caused monster PMS and put her at risk for breast and ovarian cancer. The extra neurotransmitters gave her abundant energy, enthusiasm, and drive, filling her with a sense of confidence and optimism. But they also made it hard for her to power down" (96). I too had a slow COMT. This explained my sensitivity to the roller coaster of symptoms, it explained my cysts, it explained why I was not able to find balance. It also explained why I could not handle or clear out my stress chemicals. But it also opened up something more important for me. It described why I had such buoyancy and passion. I was able to express myself as an empath and connect so well with people. Overall, my chemicals, when working right, were my gift. But too much of a good thing is a bad thing, and my body loved the high and never wanted to come down. The slow COMT loved that vigor during my younger years, but, as I aged, it was begging for the transition to a calmer, more balanced life. It craved the ability to move in and out of action and execution to rest and restoration. I was awakening to my reality for the first time in my life, and I shed buckets of tears at this realization. Through all of this information, I was finding myself for the first time, accepting who I was, and discovering the changes I would need to make to heal.

It is still very hard for me to believe that not one physician on this journey had suggested gene testing. I was sensitive to estrogen, and my body's response was to recirculate it instead of clear it, therefore creating ovarian cysts. Genes tell us so much about our story. They help us navigate the Wilderness. I wish I would have known how much this information would change my approach to my healing. Finally, something made sense, and the picture only got clearer and more connected the more I pushed for answers.

What I Wish I Knew About Epigenetics

Epigenetics is the theory that the way we eat, our stress, and our overall health impacts our genes and their expression. We can have the cancer gene and never get cancer. Or we can have the cancer gene, eat poorly, have poor gut function or metabolism issues, and get cancer. But we can determine our risk by being armed with genetic information. "The process of turning genes on and off is known as gene regulation. Gene regulation is an important part of normal development" (MedlinePlus). Bottom line, we can have a genetic predisposition but never turn that gene on if we know how to manage it. That's life-changing! It's like a puzzle that nobody had ever explained to me before. It was a major key to unlocking my personal gateway to health. I wish I would have learned about my genetic predispositions earlier in life. I could have avoided some of the things that interfered with my body's ability to handle stress and to detoxify chemicals while also being mindful of what I put in my body. This information could have given me an opportunity to be proactive in navigating my health.

I call gene testing a map or navigation tool for a reason. While many people are afraid to know if they carry a particular gene mutation, I was not willing to live that way any longer, and I knew it would be up to me to navigate my healing based on this new knowledge.

Things Get Worse Before They Get Better

In September 2021, my husband retired from serving as a chief of police. It was an exciting time for us. I was planning a big party for him as it was also his birthday, and then we were heading to Vail, Colorado, for a vacation after his celebratory event. I was thrilled about this transition after two very difficult years of him leading his team through COVID, racial tension, protests, and unimagined stress as a new chief in one of the worst times in recent history. God had him there to use every single gift that he had, and he beautifully navigated situations that very few could have handled. He was strong, patient, caring, balanced, and responsive. We had made it through. I planned a beautiful retirement party and worked hard to make the day special, and it was. Our family was there, as well as our friends and his co-workers, and I was full of energy and happiness watching life unfold before us. We were ready to enter into the best time of our lives. We had savings to enjoy life's blessings and time to enjoy each other and our families. It was time to slow down and begin the second half.

Vail could not have been more beautiful. The mountains were clear and filled with sunshine and green leaves that hung on the trees like drops of honey. I was in awe of this place. We hiked, and I even got to experience fly fishing for the first time. Being in nature made me emotional as I realized the beauty of God and all He had provided in our lives. I felt blessed and realized how fortunate we were to have this moment. Maybe, just maybe, this was the beginning of a new chapter for us and for me.

I don't know if it was the anticipation of life changing or what gripped me, but the night before our flight back home, I woke up with a sudden adrenaline rush. Something hit me hard. I was restless, anxious, and felt tense in every area of my body. I wanted to wake my husband but decided it would pass and didn't want to worry him. However, I tossed and turned all night. When we woke up to catch our flight, I was uneasy again. I felt both wired and tired at the same time. As we packed to leave, the unease became stronger. I felt a heaviness that grew more oppressive with each passing hour. My eyes were sensitive and hurt in their sockets. When we got home, I just wanted to crawl into bed. I thought maybe I was crashing from the high from all the planning. Perhaps I just needed rest. But it didn't stop. It only got worse. Everything was foggy, and I couldn't focus or function. I just wanted to sleep. I called the doctor. We did labs. A feeling of dread grew in the back of my mind as I was reminded of another time I had these same sensations. Sure enough, I had once again gotten mono. Mono is from a virus called the Epstein-Barr virus that is triggered by stress and a lack of immunity.

The first time I experienced mono was after having a horrible menstrual cycle in junior high. My bleeding was intense, and my emotions were in constant flux. I was crying, overeating, easily upset, and sensitive. I remembered all of this as my labs came in, and I felt every emotion and the heaviness from over thirty years prior. Our bodies and our cells have their own memories housed in the part of the brain that is called the hippocampus. My memories took me back to my first bout of mono, only this time there was no period, just a mass of feelings with nowhere to go. I was crashing and felt totally out of control, emotionally and physically. I couldn't think clearly, and I couldn't stop shaking. Worse, I could not find my "why" for this illness, and, for a person who craves control, not having a "why" made me feel powerless. I felt defeated, once again disappointed that joy had been snatched away from me, and all I felt was pain and exhaustion.

Faithful Dr. M. was doing her very best for me. She tested my estrogen; it was yo-yoing from 250 to 50 pg/mL and back up again. I felt every fluctuation like whiplash. We went back to the drawing board and tried everything from supplements to hormone therapy to eventually the dreaded antidepressants. This would be my second time on these drugs. What a mistake! I had been on Lexapro fourteen years prior after my issues with diet pills as I was detoxing and finding my brain unable to cope. At that time, Lexapro was a miracle drug for me. It stopped my anxiety in its tracks! It mellowed my feelings to the point of not feeling much of anything, which was okay given my stress levels. Then, one day, as I was in the car listening to the radio and my favorite song came on, I realized I felt nothing. Not one goose bump or faithful spirit of joy that once filled me as a child in my room. It was all gone, and I knew right then it was those pills. It took me about a month to wean off of them. I truly thought I would never take them again, but my desperation after that second bout of mono was so high, and my doctor was so sure I needed them, that I forced myself to fill the prescription. I started slow and low on only 5 mg and cut them in half to minimize the rush of the impact. I was hopeful that I would find a miracle in this drug and a way to stop the anxiety from controlling my life. My first night found me ruminating, full of so much adrenaline that I could chew through the walls. After seven days of hell, I had to stop them as I started to develop suicidal ideation. I was at rock bottom, holding on by a thread.

I stopped the Lexapro only to be confronted once again with another cyst. As a last-ditch effort, we tried the birth control pill, which I was told should stop the cysts from growing. Again, my tired body rejected it. I blew up like a balloon in six days. I felt helpless and hopeless. Nothing, absolutely nothing, was working. I stopped taking the pill after only seven days without any idea of what in the world I would do next. While all of this flux occurred in my body, there was a larger and unexplainable "pushing" going on around me.

A Strange Season of Reconciliation

The harder you push on something, the harder it pushes back. The transition into menopause would be no different. I continued to struggle and focused on waking up each morning and putting one foot in front of the other. I felt weak. And I was, in fact, weak. The chemical and hormonal changes had moved me into a weakened state physically, mentally, and emotionally. And this overarching weakness made me vulnerable, particularly to past traumas that were starting to resurface. And though none of us likes the feeling of vulnerability, it ultimately leads to a better place in life. I noticed that as each day passed, some radical things started to transpire that I believe at my core came to heal my soul. There was something calling to me during this time. I felt a deep yearning in my soul to reconcile things in my life that had been broken. Relationships and past hurts were screaming to be mended. Many years before I entered the perimenopause Wilderness, during my recovery from diet pills, I had met Bill Faris, a pastoral counselor, wise soul, man of God, and a man filled with discernment. He taught me so much over the years.

One of the most important things he taught me was the power of forgiveness and reconciliation. Reconciliation requires that everything has its place.

Something about this menopause transition was pushing me to reconcile my past hurts. Such healing might be the only thing we have to hold on to when we feel as if we are losing our minds. I realized something important was happening during this transition—something good, even in all the bad. It felt as though something that was bigger and stronger than the chaos was rising above me. The chaos was alive and rumbling beneath it, but there was something more powerful moving in the undercurrent of my life. I could see it, but, sometimes, it didn't seem real. I had a very hard time understanding how pain and transformation could happen in parallel. To this day, I know it was God because not one of these events would have happened outside of this season in my life.

I divorced my first husband more than twenty years ago. We always struggled to develop a good relationship after our divorce as we both blamed each other for our failed marriage. My feelings toward him were nothing short of mean-spirited and unforgiving and included an unhealthy dose of resentment. All these years later, he had become very sick with colitis, like our son, only for him, at the age of fifty-one, it was much worse. My son called me, pouring out his heart about his dad, and my heart ached with compassion. My ex-husband needed several hospital stays and urgent treatment. I found myself feeling so much pain for him and so much sadness. I was crying and praying for answers for him. I was feeling regret for being so hard, so mean, so lacking of any thread of compassion. What had happened to me? I didn't recognize myself. I had always been caring, even in the hardest of circumstances. My heart was breaking for him and his family and for my son as he began to relive every experience he had gone through with his dad. Life can be so cruel. I finally reached out to my ex-husband and his wife and told them I was praying for them and told them to hold on because God wasn't done with him yet; he had too much to fight for. We were both suffering, and my soul could finally identify with him. Suddenly I realized that a part of me I had missed was coming back to life.

I have been a sensitive person since I was a child. As I climbed the ladder of career success in my twenties and thirties, I lost sight of that little girl. I forgot about these feelings and let the driven adult take over. It was much easier to do things than to feel things. The driver loved the energy, and it always kept me in control while holding others at a distance. But during my time in the Wilderness, my sensitive heart returned and came back with a deep desire to be set free. Out of nowhere, I was reminded of one of my report cards in elementary school—a brown, torn-edged card with words that said, "Irene is sensitive to her peers." Even in third grade, there she was. Perhaps I was simply recovering who I really was, the soul I had lost with all the striving. Losing myself to find the world and coming up empty had led me back to my true nature. The child who cried with such ease, who cared so fiercely, who unashamedly sang her lungs out and felt every emotion needed to be heard. The pain of life and trauma had hit, and, one layer at a time, I had covered her up. The focused, driven, and perfectionistic persona emerged as a protector and never wanted the vulnerable child to feel again. She received the message that we had to be strong and fight forever, but I had no fight left in me. I looked in the mirror and saw the tiredness in my eyes. No more pretending, no more striving. I wanted my life back. I had begun to realize that when we condition ourselves to not feel, it's difficult to find ourselves again. It's a pressing and pulling. We don't know if we are coming or going, but we know transformation is happening, and there is no getting out of it, as scary as it might be. "You are in it now," was all I could think. I was in the ebb and flow of who I was and who God wanted me to be. He wasn't done with me.

At this same time, my son was turning twenty-five. My son owns my heart. Our relationship has not always been easy, mostly because I pushed too hard to ensure he did all the "right things" to have a successful life. If only I had realized that my recipe for success was a recipe for disaster. My son and I are so much alike that sometimes our battles felt like wars. Headstrong and focused with strong verbal skills, we could take each other down with our tongues. Creating a small version of yourself can really be rough! Our communication with each other was never easy because we both spoke over each other and never listened. After his twenty-fifth birthday dinner with his new girlfriend and my family, he came over to our house and we had the rare opportunity to be alone. As we sat together, he asked me something very vulnerable that took me aback. "Mom, why didn't you and Dad make it? Why couldn't you survive the ups and downs of marriage?" I was shocked by the question and overwhelmed by the emotions that filled my heart. How do you answer such a complicated question? I could only surmise that he had realized he was in love with his new girlfriend and wanted "better" for himself. I did too. My answer flew out of my mouth like someone else was talking. My answer was honest and the kind of truth that felt as though it had been on the tip of my tongue for years. I told him that while I realized he felt his dad had left our marriage, I had left to have an affair with my job. I also told him that in any relationship, it takes two people to make it work and two people to tear it down. I encouraged him to no longer hold only his dad accountable for our divorce. I was also at fault. My son looked up at me with tears in his eyes. He cried and asked me why I had never told him this before. I told him I never thought it was okay to admit mistakes, to humbly admit that you are not perfect, to deny yourself the freedom to come to a place of truth about yourself. He told me those were the most important words he had ever heard out of my mouth. There was a shift that night, a boulder between us that was removed. God was breaking me down to open me up one situation at a time. I was discovering myself in a way that was beyond anything I knew I was capable of. Something that only time in the Wilderness can make happen. Once there, we are so broken, so vulnerable, and so tired that we stop resisting looking at ourselves, and suddenly it doesn't feel that scary anymore. In fact, it feels scarier not to look. I was turning inside out. It was painful and liberating, but it was all around me like a blanket of emotion. I realized that without reconciliation, I could not move forward. Reconciliation of a life of pain and a desire for my heart to find healing was growing from deep within the soil of my life.

In December 2021, as Christmas neared, I was feeling nostalgic. I was thinking about my past and the father I never knew, and I found myself yearning to know what was happening in his life and, mostly, if he was okay. Why in the world, after so many years, was that on my mind? Who even cared? He never cared about me, so why would I worry about him? But the thoughts were there, and they were relentless. So again, in a hotel room, alone in Los Angeles, I picked up the phone and called the one person who could provide some answers.

My half-sister and I had met a few times over the years. My first time meeting her was when my dad drove me from Los Angeles to Sacramento to spend Thanksgiving with him and his wife. It was the first time I had seen him in over ten years. He had contacted me and asked to spend time together. I was filled with joy that the man who had rejected me wanted me back in his life. He also wanted me to meet his wife. I was hopeful that visit would be a huge turning point for us. Then, he dropped a bomb on me as the car neared the offramp to their home. Not only had he recently married, but PS., I had a sister. PPS., they both had just learned of my existence one week before my visit. Meeting the young six-year-old made me so happy. She was cute, funny, and loved meeting her big sister. Meeting her mother was another story. She answered the door in a Jack Daniel's t-shirt holding a tumbler of straight vodka in her hand and reeked of drunkenness. I was far from home, and my spirit felt fear. What was I thinking, going there to a world I knew nothing about? I made the best of it but was sad as I watched them pay more attention to their next drink than their little girl. It was clear that my half-sister was living a life that would only bring feelings of pain, rejection, and abandonment over time. I knew because I was very familiar with these feelings.

Ten years would go by before I saw her again. She came to visit me and met my family, and I loved her as much as she would let me. She was shy and had a huge smile that she hid behind. Though we enjoyed our time together, we would not see each other again until I found her on Facebook several years later when she was pregnant with twins. I was with her when her children were born; I thought we would be close. But people who don't know how to have relationships don't have them. We both had baggage, and neither one of us maintained contact.

So that night, from my hotel room in Los Angeles, I began to text her with my heart pounding. How would I explain to her why I was reaching out? So much time had gone by, so much had happened to me. What had happened to her? She was angry in response, wondering why I wanted to find my dad after so long. I didn't know how to share fifty-one years of heartache over a text. I just knew that there was something I needed to know, that maybe he was sick, or worse, dead. I needed answers.

Though she finally agreed to a call, she was angry and full of resentment. I did not know why. She seemed upset that I had reappeared after so many years. Something instantly washed over me. A wave of calm and peace. A peace beyond the comprehension of man. A love for her. A deep sadness. I realized that I recognized this person. I was her twenty years before. She was a version of me once upon a time. A broken version. I had a realization while talking to her that my perimenopause transition was driving transformation inside me. It was also the first time I realized that even in the deep heartache of my suffering, I was becoming a different person, refined by the fire. It was the first time I would see "the change" as a gift because I almost did not recognize myself or my response to her. I simply responded that I was fifty-one and going through lots of changes and seeking peace in my life. Part of that peace was making peace with my dad, letting him know I loved him and that I forgave him for a life without him. I just needed a way to get a hold of him. She told me in no uncertain terms that I might not want to do that because he had developed Alzheimer's. I paused. There was a knowing in my spirit. It was God's will that I made this call. I needed the truth. She responded that I should've expected nothing less due to all the drugs and alcohol he and her mother had done. I was silent. I told her that she sounded upset, and I understood it; she had been through a lot. She refused to give me his number, refused to allow me to connect with him. But I stayed calm. I felt as though I was having an out-of-body experience, feeling that moment with such clarity and understanding. I asked about her life, and she stated repeatedly that she was happy and successful. Like me, she had also figured out that "doing," "driving," and "pretending" would equal escape from pain. If only she had known how wrong she was. If only I could have shared fifty-one years of wisdom. But that did not happen. She left me with one sentence: "Well, I guess we are the only family we have." I told her she was right. The only thought that came to my mind was brokenness and how it is carried through generations until we choose to end the cycle. I hope this book finds its way to her. I hope she finds peace. I hope someday we can sit in the yard and laugh together. I pray for God to help her find her way to a full and happy life. She was robbed and deserves it. I deserved it too, and I desperately wanted to change the way I viewed and approached all of my life's heartbreaking circumstances but was not sure how.

Changing the way we see pain and struggle is how we rewire the brain. I began to think that maybe these pushes for reconciliation were the whole point of perimenopause turning me inside out. That this physical, spiritual, and emotional struggle was a cutting away of all that did not serve me to become who God meant me to be, but I was in the messy middle of it all. The turning inside out was shattering all my defenses, and I cried while I tried to identify who I was. Was I the driver and get-it-done girl, the person who does whatever they need to do at whatever the cost? Or was I the caring, compassionate woman who mourned the love she had missed out on? Was I upset and angry, or was I sad? Ultimately, I decided I was all of it, and it was finally pouring out of me from the vault I had kept it buried in for years. I was covered in chains. Chains that had tightened each time I was afraid of being rejected and left behind. God is in the chain-breaking business, this I now know for sure. So, while this seemingly random push toward reconciliation made no sense, it made all the sense in the world. This transition would mean doing work not only physically but emotionally and mentally. The peace would come through getting to the root of my pain regardless of how hard it would be to face it.

There was peace in knowing I had communicated with my half-sister that night. It fell over me like a blanket, and I slept better than I had in months. These kinds of experiences, these Godincidences, would continue to happen over the next several weeks. This period of reflection was constant for me. Some days, I would remember things that once brought me joy, and I would cry for the life I had forgotten about. Other days, I would remember things with such regret that my anguish felt like it would consume me. I was grieving. I would kneel on the ground and cry out to God in desperation. I kept asking "why," repeatedly and out loud. I was angry at God, angry at my situation, my brain, my health, this change. It was too much, and I didn't feel like I was strong enough to carry it all. But I have learned that for something to grow, you have to uproot the ugly messes of your past and till the soil. There is no other way.

What I Wish I Knew: The Body Keeps Score

One of the most insightful and impactful books I have ever read is *The Body Keeps the Score*, by Bessel van der Kolk, M.D. As one of the world's foremost experts on trauma, he has spent decades working with survivors of trauma. I read this book at the suggestion of my counselor midway through my perimenopause journey as I started to realize that the images in my mind and in my dreams were taking me back to the traumatic experiences of my life—the times when I felt I was lacking control or a safety net. During those times, I covered the pain and pushed hard to overcome my challenges with more work and more drive to find acceptance. But, during my time in the Wilderness, my inner child was dying to be heard and, most of all, to be reconciled. I wish I had read his book earlier in my life because it explains with so much wisdom what happens to the body and to the brain because of trauma. Trauma compromises our relationships, our ability to trust, and our immune systems. If only I had this awareness in my twenties and thirties, I might have known that there was so much more to my experiences than what I realized. My body, too, had been crying out to me during my menopausal transition, desperate for me to hear its voice, calling me to stop and look at my life, to work through my trauma, to find peace in it. "While we all want to move beyond trauma, the part of our brain that is devoted to ensuring our survival (deep below the rational brain) is not very good at denial. Long after a traumatic experience is over, it may be reactivated at the slightest hint of danger and mobilize disturbed brain circuits and secrete massive amounts of stress hormones. This precipitates unpleasant emotions, intense physical sensations, and impulsive aggressive actions. These post-traumatic reactions feel incomprehensible and overwhelming. Feeling out of control, survivors of trauma often begin to fear that they are damaged to the core and beyond redemption" (Van der Kolk 2). There is no doubt that my journey made me confront memories of my past and emotions that scared me and made me feel threatened, as well as triggered a fight or flight response that seemed irreparable.

Humans are complicated. We are a combination of DNA, experiences, and a body designed to survive. Dr. van der Kolk's book gave me logic for my emotions. If I knew what was happening, I could find a way through (despite the anguish it caused). Joyce Meyer, my favorite preacher, often says, "The only way is through." She was right.

The Bathroom Floor

I am very familiar with the bathroom floor. I find myself there when things are unbearable, and my heart is aching. I was there again as my cyst returned and pressed against my stomach, causing excruciating pain in my lower back. I knew then that there was a direct correlation between my cysts and my heartache. They grew together. So, in January 2022, I once again found myself on the bathroom floor, exposed and wounded, looking for the answer in a baptism. I wept tears of prayer for relief and for wisdom. "God, how can this anguish be worth it? I have changed so much, so why is my suffering so relentless?"

God reminded me of my earlier commitment to stop asking "why." It wasn't the point. My promise to ask the bigger question, the "what" question, echoed in my mind and soul. What was I supposed to do with all of this? Then, I heard Him say, "This has nothing to do with you and everything to do with every soul suffering like you have." It was suddenly so clear, and it felt good to have the answer, even though it was not the answer I wanted. I wanted the suffering to end. The "what" is this book you hold in your hands today. I knew I had to start writing but didn't know exactly where to start or if I even had enough energy or courage. But as God does, He took control, and what followed was the very beginning of everything that mattered. However, it would come with a pressing that I never would have expected.

The Pressing

It was February 2022, and I was miserable, unable to manage my foggy thinking and the endless hours of adrenaline and anxiety that raced through my veins. Dr. M., out of pure desperation, decided to try birth control one more time. She knew how difficult this was for me and how my body reacted to the pill, but she said it was this or Lupron (a hormone suppressant) because the only solution at this stage was to stop the estrogen from growing my cysts. My instincts were screaming, but my mind needed to rest, and I thought I needed to listen to my doctor. I visited my surgeon; he was brilliant, and I trusted him. Both doctors believed it was the right move. They hoped it would stop ovulation and, therefore, stop my cysts. So, we began with round two just before Valentine's Day. On February 14, I was wound up tighter than a drum. My husband took me to dinner. My stomach ached, but it felt less swollen. Maybe the pill was working?

The birth control pill, like most things, had an instant effect on my sensitive body. I was told to take it at night before bed, and, while I struggled to get restful sleep, I woke up feeling like a new person and was grateful that my energy was back! At 5:00 pm on the fourth day of being on the pill, I decided to relax with a hot yoga class to find my namaste. Within forty-five minutes, a strange feeling came over me, a feeling of total rage. I wanted to punch the person beside me. I was adrenaline-filled in a yoga class! I was overwhelmed and terrified at the same time. I went home to look up the side effects of the pill I was taking and came across "may cause irritability." Another website said it may cause homicidal feelings! As I read through each review, I wondered how this drug had been made safe for people. And I was frustrated that my body was once again responding to medication in such a dramatic way. It didn't feel fair. I stopped taking the pill on that day. There had to be another way to heal … God willing.

What I Wish I Knew About Suffering

As I questioned my experiences and looked for answers day after day and month after month, I became a student of scripture and psychology. I believe that God made science and that if we explore both, we find the beautiful creation of the human body, the complicated pieces, and the keys to unlock the most difficult challenges. The body, mind, and spirit are very interconnected, but, as a society, we treat symptoms of the body with little reflection on our toxic thoughts, our spirit, or our wounds. As I studied scripture, I learned a lot about suffering. Jesus suffered immensely as did His followers. His Word tells us that suffering produces character and perseverance. "We also rejoice in our sufferings, because we know that suffering produces perseverance; perseverance, character; and character, hope" (Romans 5:3–5). No doubt, I was changing as a person from the suffering. I had to keep going until the work was done.

At this time, I had started reading and listening to podcasts by Dr. Henry Cloud, a clinical psychologist and leadership expert who co-wrote the book *Boundaries*. As if God ordained it Himself, I stumbled upon another book Dr. Cloud co-authored called *How*

People Grow: What the Bible Reveals about Personal Growth. As I began to read through the book, a page opened that changed my view of my entire journey and gave me a profound sense of hope—a new hope and a deeper belief that my suffering was purposeful. "We all have coping mechanisms that cover up pain, help us deal with fear, enable us to cope with relational inabilities, and help us hold it all together. Trials and suffering push those mechanisms past the breaking point so we find out where we need to grow. Then true spiritual growth begins at a deeper level, and we are healed. Righteousness and character take the place of coping" (Cloud and Townsend 213). Like that same spirit of fear that had entered into my life when my son was sick, a spirit of perseverance walked in, a reason to believe God was changing me through my suffering. I reflected on Romans 5 again, but it had a new and deeper meaning. Perhaps the suffering was where I would find my victory.

Maybe a Miracle?

The day after stopping the pill, I woke up like nothing had happened. After seven months of each day being more difficult than the last, I felt much less anxiety. I wondered if maybe the pill was still in my system and working. Each hour, I felt more and more like myself. Energized. Focused. Active. I counted each day that went by without my heart pounding and my body shaking as a good day. I woke up with total clarity, a quiet mind, and freedom from the fear that had stalked me for years. I thought that God had given me the miracle I had been praying for and that my time in the Wilderness was finally all over. My husband noticed my energy and my consistent mood. He also thought I might be back!

Then, like always, my stomach grew and became unbearably painful. Once again, Dr. M. worked hard to find solutions and did several tests. She knew how hard I was fighting for myself, and she was right there fighting with me. What a blessing she was to me! She did another round of hormone level testing, and my estrogen was higher than ever. How that could happen to a fifty-one-year-old woman who was supposed to be approaching menopause was astounding.

With full transparency, Dr. M. told me that my fight was finally over. It was time to get my ovaries removed. "We have tried it all, Irene, nothing has worked." She called the surgeon who had removed my previous cyst and let him know it was time for the surgery that would change my entire life. But hadn't my life already changed beyond repair? It was a mess; I was a mess. I agreed to the surgery consultation.

The days continued to pass with me feeling emotionally stable, but, physically, I was swollen and unable to handle the pain in my stomach and ovaries. I prayed over and over, asking God for a word, something to hold on to. I remembered everything I read about suffering, but just like a movie that crescendos in the middle, the intensity of my situation was reaching its peak. I had scheduled an appointment with the surgeon for February 22, 2022, for the final surgical decision. While waiting for this day to come, I read the Bible and wept. There it was in black in white. Deuteronomy 2: "You have been standing at this mountain for too long." This was from the story of the Israelites who had taken forty years for an eleven-day journey. The Israelites kept showing up in my story. I needed to trust God and not let my own desire for control get in the way. I could not outrun this; it was bigger than me. I hated this truth, but it was clear that the mountain before me was my fierce will to control every situation regardless of what God wanted for me.

The days that followed before my surgery consultation were so good emotionally that I began to wonder if I had made all of this up in my head, but nobody could ignore my stomach. I looked like I was three months pregnant again, only this time the cyst pushed on my bladder and kept me up all night. Still, I felt so free from the terror of anxiety that had taken over for so long that I didn't even care if I looked this way for the rest of my life. I just wanted the mental stability to last. I slept with castor oil packs every night, which helped temporarily reduce the inflammation and pain of the ovarian cysts. Castor oil packs have been used as a folk remedy for years to reduce pain and inflammation. They have been proven to help detoxify the liver and even the lymphatic system. I would wrap myself in flannels with a castor oil pack overnight and would wake up with less bulging, only to end the day right back where I started. This was only a band-aid. I had to get real. I could no longer wear pants and found it hard to go out without feeling uncomfortable. I needed someone to talk to. I texted my two God-fearing friends letting them know I needed support. We planned breakfast for two days later.

We are wired for connection, particularly as life turns cruel and unmanageable. I showed up to the breakfast with my heart in my hands, and I spoke every word about what was happening to me. I told them that I had been praying and that I was going to tell the surgeon that after researching this kind of surgery, I only wanted one ovary removed so that my body could continue to produce some of its own hormones without fully emptying out my tank. I had done my homework and knew that a double oophorectomy was going to take me off a cliff hormonally. There was no way I could handle that level of change. I was determined to manage the surgery my way. They said it seemed logical; however, they also said we needed to pray for God's will over my situation. So, we did. Their words were like peace to my soul. I felt their love for me. I felt God's love. He was going to make a way. I just knew it.

Go Big or Go Home

I had never taken my husband to any of my medical appointments, but I felt this decision needed his input. We were scheduled to see the surgeon at 11:30 am, but we waited for thirty-five eternity-filled minutes before we were finally greeted by a nurse. She was there to discuss the specific details of what I would experience through the removal of both ovaries. I stopped her immediately, reminding her that I had not yet decided on the surgery and absolutely had not yet decided if both of my ovaries would be removed! She insisted that we go over the details and that I needed to start signing paperwork. I did not like that at all. Panic set in, and I could feel my heartbeat deep in my throat.

After signing my life away on a surgery I was not sure I even wanted, the surgeon walked in. He was a urogynecologist, which means he did bladder, pelvic, and gynecological surgeries. He was kind and compassionate, but also direct and to the point. My kind of guy! His presence said, "I know what I'm talking about" but with total humility. He was incredible. I went into a tirade about how I wanted only one ovary removed and not two. The whole praying for God's will thing was out! I explained how good the last fourteen days (yes, I was counting!) had been, how emotionally stable I was, and how badly I wanted to hold onto that feeling but could no longer handle the physical pain. "I'm so scared to crash, please don't let me crash!" He consulted my latest labs, which indicated an estrogen level of 371 pg/mL and said, "These levels won't stay like this. What you are experiencing is a high level of estrogen that is not fluctuating." The light bulb went on. That was why when I had cysts I felt stable emotionally. I was sensitive to the fluctuations, the ups and downs of the hormones. I had hormone vulnerability and sensitive estrogen receptors while also being a deeply feeling person who could not easily clear out her neurotransmitters. The clarity hit me like a two-by-four! It all finally made so much sense. But even with everything making sense, I was in total fear, knowing deep inside that this surgery could change me forever. I was promised that this would finally bring me hormone stability.

The surgeon told me that I was overproducing estrogen at high levels, which, over time, could potentially cause cancer. My husband's eyes became wide. I wanted to run out of the room. I wanted to wake up and have all of it be over. Then, he broke my heart and dashed my ambitions for a less invasive surgery: "Irene, the ovaries work separately, not together. One can produce just as much estrogen as both because they take turns producing the hormones each month during ovulation." He looked me straight in the eye and said with a firm but sweet kindness, "Irene, it's time to go big or go home; I cannot keep chipping away at your ovaries. We take both or we just wait this out." Tears streamed down my face. I felt helpless. I cried a cry of total defeat, like I had lost a battle I had been fighting for fifty-one years. I looked over at my husband as he said, "Irene, you have been chasing this for too long." I signed the papers with shaking hands on February 22, 2022—22, 22, 2 ovaries. No surprises there. I was scheduled for surgery on Monday, February 28, 2022, at 6:00 am.

The Best Sex of My Life

On the Saturday night before my surgery, I found myself in a mental battle with my decision. I told my husband we should have sex because I had read that it would be six to seven weeks until he could touch me following my surgery. But we were both exhausted and decided getting sleep was more important than having sex. I went to bed crying, feeling like my femininity and womanhood was slipping away from me. Over the previous six months, I hadn't been able to enjoy sex at all because I was often too bloated to feel sexy or too dry to enjoy it. I was desperate for intimacy with my husband again. We were always able to connect so much in this way before the Wilderness stole it all from me. I had been robbed. Moreover, I had heard many stories about women not being able to have a satisfying sex life after ovary removal. I was terrified of this. Would I lose my desire? My marriage?

As I fell asleep, I was sweating so badly I thought I was breaking a fever. Clearly, my body was in a battle with itself. I started to dream that my husband and I were having the most incredible sex ever. He was telling me it was the best sex he had ever had. I could feel every part of it in my dream. We were at a beautiful hotel with large windows all around us. I woke up. I woke him up. I told him I needed him. That night we had life-giving, soul-reviving sex. We made love. The kind that feels like an out-of-body experience. The kind that makes you feel totally alive and connected to your spouse. I was so thankful. I was also afraid. Would this be the last time I would feel this way? Was my life beginning or ending with this major decision? I didn't know who I would be when I woke up from that surgery. One thing I knew for sure was that there was no turning back.

Sunday, February 27, 2022:
The Doubting

My sleep that Saturday night was deep and refreshing. I woke up on Sunday feeling energetic and went for a long walk followed by a good weight workout. I was feeling so good that I wondered how I could even consider surgery. Why in the world was I preparing for something so dramatic, something that suddenly felt so unnecessary? Maybe my body wanted to heal on its own? Maybe I needed to be more patient, pray more? I was constantly negotiating with myself. I laid flat on my back in my garage after my workout feeling my body wanting rest. But even more than my body, my mind wanted to stop the back-and-forth of this experience. *Enough already, God, enough!*

I debated with myself about whether I should call to cancel the surgery. I wanted a sign, so I asked God for one. I needed something to help my soul find rest in this difficult decision. Then, I got one. As I walked upstairs to shower, I felt my stomach start to bloat again; the pain was there, the cyst was pushing my body over the edge. As I took each step, I felt it more acutely. Then, as I took off my clothes and walked to get a towel, I felt water dripping down my leg. I looked down to find that, while I could not feel it, I was urinating on myself. The pressure of the cyst was pushing so hard on my bladder that I could no longer control use of it. I looked hard in the mirror and convinced myself that this wasn't normal and that there was no option other than the surgery. I had asked God for an answer, and He knew it would take something that serious for me to finally surrender. I would have the surgery. My fight was over.

The rest of Sunday felt like a very short day. My husband and I had lunch at my favorite spot. He is a detail guy, and, when he is stressed, he is more "on it" than ever. He tended to everything I could possibly need to be comfortable after surgery. He honored his love language of "acts of service" then and in the trying months that followed. He made a prep tray with Tylenol, sanitary pads, Kleenex, magazines, and soothing creams. Every woman should have a husband as loving as mine, and all I could think about was how my body and mind had let him down. He was my rock. Calm and consistent. He was the only reliable constant I had left in my life. I was so thankful.

The night before surgery was hard. Despite having researched everything, my mind took me places I didn't want to go. I was scheduled for a double oophorectomy. It's a mouthful. It meant that I would be shutting down the factory, the factory that made all of my hormones, or at least almost all of them. While most women experience menopause in a natural transition, I would be, well, falling off a cliff hormonally. While they would try to patch me back together through bioidentical hormone replacement therapy (BHRT), there was no promise that it would be easy. As evening came, I received a series of audio messages, beautiful heartfelt prayers from friends as they prayed over my healing. While I listened, I cried, realizing once again how much God's love through others in our lives matters in our ability to hold on and fight. I had friends from across the country writing to me and extending their faith on my behalf. I did not realize how many people really cared. It touched me deeply. That is the secret to surviving the Wilderness. When we aren't able to rely on our own faith, we can borrow the faith of others. We can stand on their strength and belief until we believe again. That is what being a Christian is supposed to be about—to be part of a community of faith-filled people who lift you through their love for Christ, who pray for you and love on you with the love of Jesus. I realized just how blessed I was by this tribe of women in my life.

That night was long as I tossed and turned until my 4:00 am wake-up call. When I opened my eyes, I realized this was it, there was no turning back. I rolled over and realized how much pain I was in and how much I needed this surgery. I thought about all the years that had passed, all the agony, all the stress. I needed it to end one way or another. I wasn't living the kind of life God wanted for me. I was not thriving. I was surviving, and barely. A peace came over me while I got dressed and got into the car with my husband. When we arrived in the darkness of the early morning, I asked him to pray over me. He prayed a beautiful prayer asking God to heal me and allow me to have a smooth transition. I was ready to face whatever was next.

After signing in at the front desk at the surgery center, I was escorted to change into my gown. As I took off my clothes, I looked down and could hardly see my toes because of my swollen belly. The last time it had been this big was when I was pregnant with my son over twenty-four years before. I realized how tired I was, how much this was costing me. I also realized that God had carried me through the Wilderness to get to this very moment. Like it or not, it was the plan for my life. I had made peace with it.

My pre-op nurse was amazing, and when they took my blood pressure, which was 102 over 60, they asked me if it was normal for it to be this low, especially just before going into surgery. I said, "Yes because I have a community praying for me!" They asked about my activity level, and I told them I was very active and healthy. I hiked, walked, biked, and did yoga. I ate nourishing food. They promised me I would bounce back much easier than most due to my lifestyle choices. Finally, a good word!

My anesthesiologist was a jokester and said he would give me just enough anesthesia to make sure I did not help the doctor with the surgery. He said it would be the best nap I ever had and promised I would wake up without too much grogginess. My surgeon showed up serious and ready to do business. I kept wondering if he had had enough coffee; it was only 6:30 am! Had he had a good night the night before? Was he fighting with his wife? All these crazy questions filled my head. When he arrived, he asked me if I was still ready to have the surgery. I let him know that since I was urinating on myself, we were doing this! They pushed in the juice, and I fell asleep within seconds.

Scars Are for Warriors

It felt like only minutes had passed when I awoke from surgery. I could hear the nurse asking me how I felt while pushing a straw and a cup of water to my lips. I was surprisingly not very drowsy and realized that I had finally crossed over. I no longer had my ovaries. I pressed on my stomach wondering if I could feel the emptiness, but there were only a couple of bandages. Almost immediately, they were calling my husband to come pick me up. The surgery had been a success, but I never saw the surgeon, only my nurse. It felt so strange. My whole life of struggle over in three hours with twenty minutes of recovery in a surgery center. I wondered how they could push me out so fast without making sure I was okay? This is the healthcare system we are conditioned to accept. In and out for $10,000, so my bed could be taken by another patient. I was out the door with only a patch of estrogen, hoping it would "catch" my fall.

The first two days after surgery were physically exhausting. The surgeon had said it would be seven days until I could drive, walk, and do some things around the house. Though my scars were small, the fatigue was like nothing I had ever experienced before. My body was tired, and I was scared about what each day would bring. Initially, my moods were fine, and I even found myself laughing with my mom and aunt when they came to visit. I was sore and tired but felt more like myself. I don't usually nap, but I needed to lie down a lot more often during my recovery. I could walk to my bedroom with some help only to collapse on the bed to rest. I received flowers, calls, and even a new pair of comfortable joggers from a client, which made me smile. Maybe my oophorectomy was everything everyone had promised … maybe it *was* my healing. The Wednesday after Monday's surgery, my whole family showed up at my house; we made tacos and had a wonderful day. I was so pleased with my recovery, I thought I might be Superwoman. My mom could not believe how uplifted my spirits were. She was sure I had done the right thing and had prayed over me for this miracle for years. I had started my estrogen patch the minute I had gotten into the car after surgery and was hopeful it would keep my levels from dipping too far down as things shifted. I also took progesterone nightly, which helped me sleep. I felt stable emotionally despite the fatigue and the soreness, so I assumed everything was working the way it was supposed to. Then, things shifted, again.

One night, as I rested in bed, I had a call from a good friend of mine. She had a hysterectomy eight years before my surgery. She told me to not be surprised if I unexpectedly found myself crying for no reason as the days passed. Her message must have been a prediction of what I would experience next. Seven days after surgery, I woke up feeling fine, had my breakfast as usual, and sat outside to get some sunshine. Suddenly the tears came for absolutely no reason just as she had forewarned. Not really crying but sobbing. It was as though someone had turned the water faucet on, and I could not switch it off. I didn't understand it all. I had read about hormone shifts, and I had experienced them in many extremes, but this felt different. I felt like a shell caught in a wave that was crashing to the ground. I would cry into my husband's arms, I would cry into my pillow, in the shower, day and night. I felt as though my body was grieving. It was surreal.

I was reminded that someone once told me that for something to come to life something else must die. My new emotional experience was grief. I was grieving everything that was gone. My ovaries, my drive, my stability, my old self. I called my friend. I thanked God for her. She assured me it would be okay and reminded me that my body had been through major trauma. She also told me it would take a year to feel fully healed. I cried harder. But hearing her voice, even though the words were piercing, made me feel less alone. Someone else had gone through this and survived. I needed to keep my eyes on this truth.

Nobody really understands the way a body is going to respond to surgical menopause; it is unique for every woman. It is not like natural menopause. I was no longer a full body functioning like other people function. I had what some have termed a "prosthetic hormonal system." Just like a prosthetic leg, it's not real. It was as close as science could get to real, but it was not *my* natural God-given hormonal system. I was patched back together with hormones that were simply not mine. My natural operating system was shut down, and I had to hope to feel the way I used to feel but with an "artificial" hormone system. Just like a computer on force quit, I had to reboot. But it didn't feel or work the same. It was different, and my whole body and brain knew it. It was at that moment I realized that the symptoms of my surgery were affecting every single cell in my body, my brain, and my neurotransmitters. My sudden lack of my own estrogen was destroying me—body, spirit, and mind. My OCD returned with a vengeance and had me wondering if I was truly mentally ill. It held on to my mind daily, never letting me out of its grip. "Increasing evidence suggests estrogen and estrogen signaling pathway disturbances across psychiatric disorders. Estrogens are not only crucial in sexual maturation and reproduction but are also highly involved in a wide range of brain functions, such as cognition, memory, neurodevelopment, and neuroplasticity" (Hwang et al. Abstract). If I thought it was bad before, adjusting to this was going to be like walking through fire. My mind kept telling me that I should have never had the surgery. Nobody, I mean nobody, prepared me for any of this. I was (and still am) completely dumbfounded by the lack of research, education, and awareness on this topic. That is part of the motivation for writing this book—to educate people and help them feel less invisible, make informed choices, and ask the right questions.

I also wish I'd known how important time and community were going to be for my healing. Time is a healer. But time on the surgical menopause journey is both a friend and an enemy. Days bleed into each other, and the healing decides when and how fast it will come. My mind had to patiently wait while my body identified how to function with a new system. My saving grace was my healthy body, my good eating habits, and my supplement regimen. Without these fundamentals, honestly, I don't know how I could have managed. My research, education, and every bit of knowledge I had acquired served me during recovery. But there was still so much I felt like I didn't know.

One day, as I laid in bed, I found a surgical menopause website on Facebook called the Surmeno Connection. It consists of more than nine thousand women with stories, helpful hints, knowledge, and, most importantly, their experiences with surgical menopause. I cannot express how thankful I am for every woman who was willing to share her story and every word of hope I was blessed with when I had none. Deprivation had turned to abundance. A community of women with a shared experience was everything during this transition. I had been scared—not just of the surgery ramifications— but scared to take a deep look at myself and admit that I wasn't perfect, admit I didn't have all the answers, and, ultimately, admit that I was weak physically and emotionally. I was scared that if I admitted this, nobody could handle it … that nobody could help me … that I would suffer alone. I believe many women fear revealing that we're crumbling inside because we're expected to make everyone else feel okay first and foremost. I'm here to say that it's okay not to be okay and strength is in finding a community, a therapist, or a friend to be vulnerable with or to be vulnerable with God. It is part of the healing. I also believe that there is beauty in looking inward. I had to find myself again, but it felt so dark. A new level of darkness in another kind of wilderness. I learned that looking inward to get to my best life meant I had to face opposition from Satan himself.

The Serpent and the Water

What I am writing will be hard to believe. It's hard for me to believe. The Saturday following my surgery, I fell fast asleep as my body needed a whole new level of rest. The kind of sleep that resembles passing out cold. I was going back to work the following Monday and was worried about whether I was ready. My external incisions were healing well, but daily tasks like showering and washing dishes remained difficult. In my deep sleep, I began to have a wildly vivid dream. I was in our home, and our kids were small. There was a large serpent winding its way around our house, and I was desperately trying to get the kids out of the house. I panicked and was crying, but they wouldn't move. The serpent slithered its way toward me, and I felt its damp skin on mine. It was circling me. I was going to die.

Suddenly, I was jolted from my sleep by my husband who jumped out of the bed and flew across the room saying there was a snake on him. I cried hard and begged him to hold me. I had no words. I could not explain it. How was it possible that we were having the same dream? That night, I realized that I was about to be in a battle with the Serpent who was determined to attack my physical and mental weakness. I explained my dream and he explained his. We were both in shock that we had experienced the Serpent together but separately.

I tried to shake it off, but it took a full day to recover from how real it all seemed, how strange it was. The very next night as I slept, I had a second dream. I was in a car, but the car was a boat and was quickly approaching water. It ended up in the water, which rose around me up to my neck. Again, I was sure I was going to die. I asked the captain, whose face I could not see, if we were going to drown. He said, "No, you will never drown; I won't let you." The boat lifted above the water's surface; we were skating over it with ease. I woke up soaked in sweat wondering if my life had turned into a movie. I soon realized that God was reassuring me that He was walking with me and would never leave me, regardless of my fear or the aggressions against me by the Enemy. His promise was bigger, and His faithfulness was true. He was my captain.

He *Knows*

For months before my surgery, my husband had been planning a trip to the mountains to go fishing with his dad, but he was scared to leave me. To be honest, I was scared too. Would I be able to get around okay? What if I couldn't cope and needed him? He was my soldier, not willing to give up on me or stop seeking to understand what made no sense, even to me. Just being there, holding me while I cried when I knew how powerless he felt watching all of this happening to me, made me feel safe. But he needed the break, and, deep inside, I knew I needed to start to rely on my own strength with God's help. It was time I rediscovered the strong, independent woman I had once been. So, I said goodbye and cried the moment he left.

I tried to distract myself with some TV, but the hospital drama I was watching only triggered my fears, doubts, and frustrations about my recovery. I felt like my battle was a lifetime prison sentence. The fatigue was the worst. It came and went in waves. They had said that was normal, but it didn't feel normal. My passion and zest for life were gone, and I felt doomed as if it would never return. I was starting to lose touch with reality from the fogginess and fatigue. I would wake up praying that the hours of energy would get longer and those of fatigue would get shorter. I prayed I could work again with zeal, to live my calling, to change the world. I had always wanted to change the world. I had once believed I could. After my surgery, I was not so sure. One day, I took a walk to revive my body and mind. As I stepped into the sunshine and looked up to the sky, two words came over me so loudly that they could not be ignored.

"I *know!*" I kept hearing the words over and over as if my body was speaking to me. I kept asking God what it meant and felt His warm embrace and spirit speaking to me. He assured me that my body knew how to heal and that I needed to be patient. The decision I made at that moment would be the decision that would anchor me in the wild of all the storms that were to come. It was the decision to *believe* and *trust* God even though nothing I was experiencing suggested that it made any sense. Like Job, who was tested and tried by losing his health, children, and wealth, I would not let go of God. We were going to do this together. So, I asked Him, "Why these words? What are you telling me?" In my heart, I heard His spirit say two profound things: "I *know* because I *am*," and "I created your body to be whole." It was the clearest message I had ever received from God.

Christians believe that God came to Earth in the form of a man to experience life as we know it. To *know* what it is like to have joy, compassion, and love but also to experience pain, suffering, and extreme anguish. His death on the cross for me was the culmination of that experience and also my freedom. God knew what I was going through and had experienced pain far greater than my own. He experienced the anguish to free me and the world. God had turned bad into good. Could that be what He was trying to do for me? Was there truly a purpose in all of this? I received a second message through scripture as I was studying and praying: "For you created my inmost being, you knit me together in my mother's womb. I praise you because I am fearfully and wonderfully made" (Psalm 139: 13–14). This was the second part of the "I *know*" message. My body had been made through God's perfect love. I just needed to find my way home through this change. It would not be easy, but it would be possible. That was His promise to me.

"The Change"

Perimenopause is defined as the time *before* a woman stops having a menstrual cycle. During this time of life, estrogen and progesterone fluctuate radically. It's like the body wants to have a last hurrah before it stops, but there is no way to expect when it will be up from the high estrogen or down from the low. Most women don't realize that progesterone declines faster than estrogen during this time, and progesterone is the calming hormone that helps us feel centered and at ease. This roller coaster can cause mood swings, depression, anxiety, weight gain, extreme irritability, and vaginal dryness as our bodies struggle to manage the onset of "the change." These erratic fluctuations feel extreme for hormonally-sensitive women, while others feel nothing. Sometimes perimenopause or other endocrine issues can temporarily halt menstrual cycles. For eighteen months during perimenopause, I was so stressed that I burned through my adrenal system to the point that my body focused only on survival and paused my menstrual cycle.

Menopause, however, is the true end of menstruation, the time when "the factory" finally shuts down. It is defined as twelve months without a menstrual period. Whoever coined the term "the change" for menopause was a genius. The ovaries stop producing progesterone, estrogen, and testosterone. It's a permanent alteration to our bodies. It's a new normal. A book that supported me during early menopause was *It's Your Hormones*, by Geoffrey Redmond, M.D., which covers hormonal vulnerability at length. It was an awakening for me. He discussed how some women are more hormonally vulnerable to "the change" than others and are more susceptible to symptoms like mood changes, hair loss, insomnia, weight gain, hot flashes, night sweats, irritability, anger, depression, and anxiety. Moreover, for some women, as we age, it becomes more difficult to manage these changes. The body is a system that includes mind, body, and spirit. My experience during "the change" taught me the power of working with all three. There were many bumps along the way, but eventually my body found homeostasis once I gave it all the things it needed.

What I Wish I Knew About Surgical Menopause and Its Effect on the Endocrine System

There is nothing natural about surgical menopause. I wish I would have understood this at a much deeper level before surgery. I wish I would have spoken to women who had experienced it. I wish I would have been more educated. Natural menopause means our body adjusts slowly. While still difficult and challenging, it rhythmically finds its new normal. Women who have natural menopause still make some of their own hormones through adipose tissue (fat) and their adrenals, which helps to compensate as their ovaries slowly shut down.

But in surgical menopause, one major piece of the feedback loop in the endocrine system shuts down completely overnight. Once the ovaries, which are as much a part of the endocrine system as the reproductive system (we tend to only consider them in their reproductive context), are gone, the body is left without its most precious hormones that give it strong bones, a good heart, a focused brain, sex drive, strong metabolism, and energy. How can we expect our bodies to feel "normal?" Our estrogen is so important for our brain, heart, and bones. It is like lubricant to our joints. It makes our serotonin come alive and our dopamine sing. Our testosterone gives us sexual vitality and muscle tone. Our progesterone balances our nervous system and helps create GABA to balance estrogen. Imagine all of this is suddenly gone. It means that every other part of our endocrine system has to readjust, instantly. Additionally, like a total cascade of impact, this major transition puts pressure on many other body systems.

What I Wish I Knew About Hormone Management

I wish I would have realized that the body sends signals as we age—whispers that get louder when unattended. Hormones are powerful messengers—we should get used to listening to them as early as possible. Hormone fluctuations are at the center of "the change" and trigger many uncomfortable, painful, even terrifying physical, mental, and emotional symptoms (as I describe in detail later). These symptoms can start in perimenopause or menopause itself. Be careful to not ignore or push through them. Being proactive with your menstrual health as early as your twenties and thirties can dramatically impact the later stages of life in both how you age and how you experience perimenopause and menopause. It is imperative to learn about hormones and their effects on your body as they change. Understand your biochemistry, get the right lab work, and gain a deep understanding of what is happening in your unique body. Getting the right tools to manage your body's impending changes can save you from debilitating symptoms. Hormone management is the first step ... the base layer ... the bare minimum for caring for yourself through perimenopause and menopause. For those who need to undergo surgical menopause, I cannot stress enough how important it is to do research, talk to others who have experienced it, and become aware of the options. I was unprepared for how much surgical menopause would change my life. If this is your only choice, get prepared. Identify how to manage your hormones post surgery and how to support your nutrition, adrenals, thyroid, and overall lifestyle. Empower yourself in advance so that you are armed with knowledge to move toward healing.

But don't stop with hormone management. I can say without question that hormones alone did not heal me. I only found truly effective healing when I broadened my scope, engaged functional medicine practitioners, and treated the systems-based conditions that were underlying the symptoms.

What I Wish I Knew About Doctors

It is almost impossible to find an integrated approach from one doctor. I had the best team, but I leveraged each one on my own to put the puzzle pieces together. This included a naturopath, a menopause specialist physician, and a doctor of osteopathic medicine. I wish I would have had resources like my practice to ease the financial burden of chasing my symptoms through specialists.

Most traditional medical doctors are trained to find solutions to problems based on *symptoms*. Western medicine treats the problem using labs to identify the issues to then leverage drugs to treat our physical and mental ailments. That was Dr. M.'s role. Her speciality in menopause management with hormones has, to this day, been invaluable to my health. But Dr. M. knew I wanted a broader team that included functional medicine practitioners—those who embrace a systems-oriented model; she understood I needed to dig to the root causes and get beyond basic hormone management; and she supported every step with love and kindness. According to the Institute for Functional Medicine, "[F]unctional medicine takes a comprehensive approach to prevention, health, and well-being; treats root causes of disease; and restores healthy function through a personalized patient experience." I wanted to uncover and manage the root causes of my challenges at the systems level beyond just treating the symptoms.

I first learned about systems theory in my graduate program. Little did I know how relevant it would be to my healing journey more than a decade later. I studied Peter Senge's work, particularly his focus on systems theory, for my final thesis paper as part of my master's degree in organizational leadership. The core theme of Senge's systems theory is that everything that happens influences something else in a nonlinear way. His book, *The Fifth Discipline*, sits on my shelf marked-up and dog-eared after years of study: "The key to seeing reality systemically is seeing circles of influence rather than straight lines. This is the first step of breaking a reactive mindset that comes inevitably from linear thinking. Every circle tells a story. By tracing the flows of influence, you can see patterns that repeat themselves, time after time, making transitions better or worse" (75). This is systems thinking, and it is how we need to view menopause if we truly want to find balance. It's not simple, it's not one or two things. It's many things working in a feedback loop of information to your brain and body. It includes gene expression, detoxification pathways, methylation, gut health, trauma healing, prayer, mindset, and hormone levels. I talk to so many women that "chase" their hormone levels, never realizing that a broken part of another piece of the system is what actually may be causing their problem. Again, I only know this to be true because of my own desperate journey to find answers.

There are very few systems thinkers or practitioners working in the field of medicine, which is how my decision to become a menopausal educator and certified hormone practitioner was inspired. Women going through perimenopause and entering menopause were suffering but given only band-aids to fix their immediate symptoms, not to improve the underlying health of their systems. My friends were quitting their jobs, and my family members were depressed. Don't misunderstand: I love doctors and have been blessed with great physicians. But I had become intolerant of the lack of information and the lack of education available to women who wanted to help themselves. I was interested in causality, and, eventually, I learned enough to help myself by becoming empowered to ask the right questions, push for the right tests, and insist on the right hormones based on my labs and knowledge of what I learned my body needed to thrive. My faith also reinforced that God made us to understand ourselves, our systems, and the root causes of our problems. We are made to listen to the whispers of our spirits, our minds, and our bodies to find our way to wholeness. I was so convinced of this at this point in the journey that I knew for sure it had to be my message, what I could leave on this Earth ... my purpose.

The Symptoms

I wish I could say that managing my post-surgical menopause changes were smooth; instead, I almost immediately started to have the symptoms that many women experience.

Healing is not linear. Let me say it again, healing is not linear. I had been told this many times by various practitioners. I know it's true. I had days post-surgery when I felt okay and even had some energy only to be followed by hours of exhaustion and anxiety. I will do my best to describe my symptoms. I also know that while some of these symptoms are related to surgical menopause, they are also related to menopause in general. The difference is surgical menopause comes with the unique challenge of zero ramp-up time to transition. It is "the change" on steroids. Please note that it does not matter if you had surgical menopause or are going through natural menopause. If you are hormonally vulnerable to the changes, you may experience this kind of suffering. Persevere. You will see the fruits of your fight, but you need to learn what your symptoms mean, how they are "speaking" to you, and then what to do about them.

The symptoms of perimenopause, menopause, and surgical menopause are wide and ever changing. Every woman will feel differently as her body starts to shut down ovarian function and slowly makes less hormones or dramatically cuts them all off due to surgical menopause. There is no way to know until we go through it what we will experience, which makes it all that much harder to prepare for. The following are my personal experiences. I'm sure there are others not listed here. We are all very different and experience this transition in our own unique way. It goes back to the intricacy of the Creator and what He created. We are indeed uniquely woven together in our mother's womb. While beautiful, it is what makes this journey so hard to manage without proper coaching and without the help of a good medical team. Ultimately, we are responsible for our own well-being.

Joint Pain

Estrogen is a major lubricator for the joints and is anti-inflammatory in the right dosages. As we enter menopause and lose estrogen, we lose this benefit. About three months into my recovery, it became hard to exercise without pain in the evenings that sometimes kept me awake for hours. I was sore and constantly trying to stretch my legs to keep my blood flowing. My legs would ache in the mornings when I woke up. Eventually, I developed extremely painful arthritis in both of my hips, which, in many ways, felt like another blow to my recovery. I loved to exercise, and it always lifted my soul. Without it, there was something else to grieve, another loss. Though I found supplements to ease the pain, ultimately, I had to realize that my body wanted calmer, more grounding movement. Yoga, Pilates, and walking eased my pain but, more importantly, eased my mind. I also learned how to strengthen my core and back to support my hips. I read books on natural therapies for healing arthritis and realized food could be medicine. So, I added turmeric and extra anti-inflammatory foods like broccoli and kale to my diet while increasing my intake of vitamins like selenium and CoQ10. Finally, I learned estrogen can lessen the effect of our thyroid and cause our joints to ache. Once I was finally able to find the right doses of estrogen and thyroid medication, I was able to minimize my arthritic flares.

Brain Fog

Being on top of my game has been an asset for me throughout my life. I was a closer, a person who could achieve anything they set their mind to. I felt safe in this role, sure of myself and my abilities. When I started menopause, I lost my clarity. My brain became so foggy after my surgery that I often felt like it was somewhere in outer space and disconnected from my body. This made me question everything about myself. Would I ever come back? Was this the start of dementia? It was terrifying for my Type A mentality. I was fearful that I would no longer have the cognitive ability or energy to work. I felt hopeless. Fortunately, I had Dr. M. in my corner. She reassured me that as my estrogen patch kicked in, I would see clearly again and my brain would turn on. Estrogen, she said, is highly responsible for brain function, and hormone replacement would ease this symptom over time. "Estrogen improves cerebral blood flow. In women who have extremely low estrogen levels because of illness or surgery, their blood-flow patterns resemble those of patients with mild to moderate Alzheimer's. In one study, it was found that administering estrogen reversed these detrimental blood-flow changes and restored a normal pattern after only six weeks" (Bluming and Tavris 141). Dr. M. was right. As the days went on and my body adjusted, the fog lifted. We added testosterone in small amounts, which also helped my brain and energy levels immensely. "Testosterone increases libido, improves mood, lessens depression, preserves memory, maintains and promotes muscle mass and strength, decreases body fat, increases exercise tolerance, protects against cardiovascular disease, improves cholesterol, maintains bone density, prevents osteoporosis, prevents tendon and joint degeneration, and maintains skin tone" (Hawkins 30). Needless to say, this hormone not only improved my brain fog, but it improved my vitality!

Hot Flashes and Night Sweats

This is often a major complaint of most women as they enter menopause or after surgery. The first few weeks after my surgery, at different times of the day, it felt as if the heater went on in the house at a hundred degrees. I remember looking down at the couch convinced someone had set it and me on fire. I would wake up with the sheets so wet I had to change my clothes. The heat would start at my feet and crawl up my neck, throwing me off balance and causing my heart to race. I would feel the sweat dripping down my neck and wonder if others thought I had just run a marathon. I can now say with happiness that this symptom is gone. Estrogen loss creates an imbalance in the body's hypothalamus, which is responsible for temperature regulation. "Triggered by falling estrogen and rising FSH [follicle-stimulating hormone], [hot flashes] tend to become more frequent as we approach our final period. That is the time when estrogen levels are the lowest and FSH levels are the highest" (Northrup 159). The heat I felt was my body trying to cool itself down. Hot flashes and night sweats can be handled with appropriate hormone therapy but require proper doctor support and care.

Irritability

As my body got deep into the perimenopausal transition, I experienced an overwhelming feeling of edginess and irritability. Like my skin was crawling. The simple sound of my husband chewing his food would fill me with rage. I knew this was not normal and, in fact, irrational, but that did not matter to my emotional response. I felt no control over the absolute anger that would take over for the dumbest reasons. I felt badly about these overwhelming reactions.

All I wanted was to be alone, to disappear until I could stabilize and be "normal" again. This irritability was truly a response to my estrogen going sky high and then down too low for my brain to handle. Knowing that made it a bit easier, but until I finally crossed over to menopause after surgery, this symptom regularly reared its ugly head.

Anxiety

Because I suffered from OCD for decades, I was already familiar with the demon of anxiety. But it came on ten times stronger during perimenopause and surgical menopause. It would grip me so hard that I thought I should admit myself into a psychiatric facility. Simply watching a scary movie made adrenaline rush through my veins. My nervous system was insanely sensitive. Any amount of stress or change in my hormone levels felt like I was touching a hot stove. I had zero tolerance. My levels would spike, and I could feel my entire system shake. I was crawling out of my skin before the surgery, and—I need to be very honest—it took almost twelve full months for the anxiety to go away after the surgery. As the days and months went by, I adjusted, and the hours of anxiety became every other day, then once a week, and finally disappeared. It was as if my body was learning how to downregulate the need for adrenaline, and I was forever resisting my need for speed in life. I had to surrender; there was no other choice. I needed to find myself again, but without deep understanding and self-management, it never would have happened. I truly believe that healing my anxiety was part miracle and, in large part, my own education, advocacy, and sheer will to heal.

Nobody should live this way, but our healthcare system is not patient enough, nor does it give women enough support to try different methods or amounts of hormone, adrenal, supplement, or thyroid therapy to meet our individual needs. Doctors don't have time to teach patients how to work on their nutrition, stress management, and lifestyle. At Meno Coaching, we hear about this lack of education all the time. No one discussed with me the importance of knowing how I was metabolizing hormones, methylating, or digesting food and clearing out toxins. I had to do endless hours of research to educate myself on how the entire physiological system worked! A body in dysregulation feels unsafe; it feels fear. Fear drives anxiety. Fear was also the spirit I had received when my son was sick. Fear enters our soul, but, let there be no doubt, it is also stored in every cell creating dysregulation and inflammation in the body and the brain. I made the decision to wrestle it to the ground. I woke up one day and said, "No matter what, I am not giving in to this until I am healed." It took many different strategies while working with my body's entire system, my lifestyle management, and self-compassion to create a safe environment for my body. Anxiety is a symptom of a body out of balance and, therefore, brain circuits misfiring. This is very common during "the change," but it's rarely discussed by professionals.

Estrogen loss, once again, was the culprit of this symptom—but in an indirect way. Because estrogen is as much a part of the endocrine system as it is the reproductive system, its sudden disappearance wreaked havoc on my adrenals. The adrenal glands produce DHEA, cortisone, and estrogen among other hormones. DHEA is produced first and triggers the adrenals to make estrogen. Since I no longer had my ovaries to produce estrogen, my DHEA spiked in an attempt to force my adrenals to create estrogen. But despite its efforts, it made me feel worse as my adrenals could not handle the spikes. My DO explained that my adrenals were essentially tapped out and sluggish due to years of abuse. They couldn't respond to compensate for the loss of my natural estrogen. And because DHEA and cortisol work in the inverse of each other to stay in equilibrium, as my DHEA skyrocketed, my cortisol fell, causing the entire system to malfunction. I had a constant feeling inside that I was hanging by a thread and was sensitive to stress, exercise, and the slightest conflict or work issue. My DO said my nervous system was in fight-or-flight mode and needed to find its way back to balance. What became clear was that my lack of ability to manage my stress all my life had now caught up with me. Christiane Northrup, author of the must-read book *The Wisdom of Menopause*, explains: "The two-thumb size adrenal glands secrete three key hormones that help us with many of the stresses and burdens of life. However, if a woman has lived for a long time with the perception that her life is inescapably stressful, or if she is chronically ill, then chances are she has asked too much of her adrenal glands and has not given them enough time to replenish themselves. Not surprisingly, EBV [Epstein-Barr virus] and other viruses thrive on the stress hormones produced by the adrenals, so many women with adrenal problems also have thyroid problems" (148). This was my story! I was chronically stressed most of my life. I had been diagnosed with the Epstein-Barr virus years before and had thyroid issues. Why didn't anyone connect the dots?

Suicidal Ideation

This one is hard to write. Full transparency, I felt shame in writing it and then realized this meant it was crucial to include. I had four terrifying episodes of this horrific experience. Each time I had a major change in my hormone levels or made changes in my estrogen patch dose or my thyroid medicine, it would come over me like a wicked oppression. I also realized that it had happened when I was sick with the flu and when I had mono. I put the pieces together after getting COVID when the darkness came over me like a black veil for two hours that felt like years. It was so intense that I researched "COVID and the brain" and learned that the body's response to healing from illness can cause the brain to become inflamed and trigger symptoms of depression. My visceral intuitive feeling to avoid antidepressants was right—my body just needed to adjust to the inflammatory healing response.

Let me be clear, I did not want to die. Rather, I wanted to stop the pain. I wanted to escape my body. It was horrific. Through countless conversations with other surgical menopause patients, I learned that many of them also had experienced suicidal ideation. They confirmed that it was, in fact, hormonal and an inflammatory response in my brain.

Despite this knowledge, I cried out in anguish as I waited for my body to adjust to the new hormonal system. I began to realize that, after surgery, I was now living in a "patched-together" system. I held on to God because He was all I had. I begged Him for mercy. Each time, He gave me His mercy. Eventually, I learned how to read exactly what my body needed and how to balance my symptoms and my therapies. My body arrived at homeostasis, but not without incredible courage, grit, tears, prayers, and effort. If this sounds like you, know that you are not alone. There is help available with the right therapies, community, and support of good coaches, doctors, and therapists. It is why I started Meno Coaching.

The Very Dry Desert of Sex

Intimacy in any marriage is so important. It keeps us connected emotionally and physically. I had always enjoyed this part of my marriage. Entering menopause changed this dramatically. Six weeks after surgery, I was told it was okay to engage in sex again. I feared having pain, but so badly needed to feel close to my husband. My soul ached for him. During our first sexual intercourse after surgery, I kept thinking about the inside of my body and my wounds, and I wasn't able to be in the moment with him or share the experience with him. The walls of my vagina felt thin and weak, like what I can only describe as a desert. It was so painful. I was told it would get better, but I didn't know if that was true, and I was heartbroken. Everything I had feared was coming true. I was a broken toy. I no longer felt sexy. Finally, after two months of pain, I called Dr. M. Beautiful, sweet Dr. M.! My sage in the Wilderness. "No problem!" she said. "I will fix this!" She prescribed an estradiol-based vaginal cream that works primarily on the lining of the vaginal walls to increase lubrication. She promised that in three weeks things would be different. This help alone was worth every dollar I ever paid her! Three weeks later, I had the most incredible sex with my husband followed by my very own orgasm. I cried, but this time with joy. I was okay; we were okay. I was not broken. I was still a woman. Thank you, God.

Depression

The demon of depression is very real for many women suffering through menopause. It is very common and not always easily treated with antidepressants. Medicine can help some women with symptoms, but others report no relief or feel worse. I encountered this new-to-me demon of depression immediately after my surgery while I adjusted to BHRT and a new, totally unnatural operating system. It was harrowing and oppressive. Without my own estrogen to make serotonin and dopamine, my hormone receptors felt starved. My mind became weak, and my stress increased in response, causing a continuous loop of depression. DHEA, testosterone, thyroid, and cortisol hormones also all play roles in mood management and warding off depressive episodes. While my hormones stabilized from BHRT, I also began managing my nutrition, my gene mutations, my gut issues, and my stress levels. Then, my depression completely ceased. It truly proved how much these feelings are the brain's and body's way of screaming for balance. It probably would have been much easier to take a pill, and, if they worked for me, I may have done so, but God knew I could trust Him to heal me and help me find my way to wholeness if I listened to my body's cry for help.

Migraines

I had never experienced a migraine in my life until surgical menopause. I thought they were just bad headaches until my head felt as if it might explode. I experienced them in the beginning of my BHRT estrogen dosing while we were trying to find the hormonal sweet spot. Migraines were a popular topic on Facebook's Surmeno Connection page. It became clear that my migraines were a response to estrogen fluctuations. At the suggestion of many of the women on the page, I began to track all my symptoms to identify when and why I was getting them. I quickly saw patterns; I was getting fluctuations during estrogen patch changes. I researched how patches work and learned that they move estrogen into the bloodstream slowly on day one and then peak before they normalize. I had to change my patch twice a week. Many women suggested overlapping patches for three to six hours to avoid fluctuations. That was game changing!! It worked! Not one more migraine after overlapping my patch for four full hours. Many of the women on the page also noted that changing the patch every three days created more stability in dosing and positively impacted their moods. Dr. M. and I talked about it, and she agreed. Another tweak that proved to be just what I needed. I was gaining ground and finally winning.

Hormone Fluctuations

We have three kinds of estrogen: estrone (E1), estradiol (E2), and estriol (E3). Estrone is the main hormone made after menopause. It is made from adipose tissue or fat, which is often why, at menopause, we gain weight and our bodies make fat—to produce extra estrogen. Estrone can also be converted into estradiol. Estradiol is the strongest of the three hormones. Its main function is to mature and maintain the reproductive system. It is the one that must be balanced with progesterone during menopause. Thus, it is the hormone that impacts women most dramatically during menopause because it drops to almost zero. Estriol is associated with pregnancy and is increased during this time by the placenta. It helps the body prepare for the delivery of a child.

While I suffered from too much estrogen my whole life, I was unprepared for the management necessary with BHRT. There are many different delivery methods: patches, shots, pellets, and pills. It's very important to understand that everyone responds differently to each of these methods. It gets very complicated. Finding the best method is essential but only happens through trial and error and with the support of a qualified doctor who is willing to look at your whole system. Patches were my choice, but they are a lot of work. Every doctor said I would feel fine so long as I got enough estrogen at a consistent level. Only one doctor was willing to be brutally honest with me. She said, "Irene, your body needs to heal, it needs time, you have been through so much." She was right. Lab tests every six weeks, while helpful, did not provide enough regular information to guide my optimal dosages. I was desperate for reliable data more often. I had heard that the Mira fertility tracker app (miracare.com), which was originally designed to help women get pregnant by testing hormone levels and ovulation, was also being marketed for menopause since its urine test kit sticks could measure estrogen and progesterone levels at any time. This was life changing for me. I checked my estrogen levels daily to see if I needed further support through estrogen gel in addition to my patch. The app allowed me to track the ebbs and flows of my estrogen levels and my symptoms. It was incredible to have this critical information at my fingertips. More importantly, it gave me some control over a very uncontrollable situation. I quickly noticed that heat, working out, and added stress diminished the effectiveness of my patch and sometimes required that I apply a little extra estrogen gel. Thankfully, Dr. M. worked carefully with me to fine tune my delivery method as I tracked my symptoms. I learned very quickly that I needed to listen to the whispers of my body and my intuition along with sound and reliable information. I also had to be patient as my body adjusted to absorbing and utilizing this new delivery method. Patience during the period of fluctuations and adjustment post surgery takes much more resilience than I ever thought possible. Many days, I felt like giving up, but, by the total grace of God, I pressed on.

Lab Tests Are Necessary Pieces
of the Puzzle

My healing has been the result of a combination of things, most importantly me at the center fighting for every bit of ground. It was God's power working within me that gave me strength during the moments where I thought the battle was going to take me down permanently. The pieces of this healing puzzle are complex, but when we are in tune with our body and educate and empower ourselves through data, support, and faith, we can heal. The puzzle does come together to reveal the full picture. Most physicians can only offer some of our puzzle pieces to each of us because they specialize in only one or two areas of the whole picture. From there, we need to piece together our puzzle as customized to each of our individual needs. That is where this gets complicated and why I created Meno Coaching, which has the breadth and depth of resources (beyond what individual health practitioner specialists can offer) to guide this difficult process. Even the best doctors cannot help us if we don't help ourselves, if we aren't willing to fight for ourselves. And believe me, we have to fight. The only way is through.

After my surgery, I initially believed that the symptoms I was facing were going to be my way of life. I was resigned and told God as I prayed that even if He did not heal me, I would walk with Him daily to cope with them. I found some resolution: no matter what, I was going to live, even if I would not find full freedom on Earth from my struggles. Something about that prayer calmed me down. I remembered Peter Senge's quote: "The harder you push, the harder the system pushes back" (58). My pushing was not helping. In fact, it was causing more stress to my mind and my body.

One morning, I pulled out all my old files—over a thousand pages of more than a decade of lab work, saliva tests, and genetic tests. I started to review the files, analyzing the patterns of all the mess I had in front of me. Instead of pushing back against my symptoms, I was going to become educated about the story they were telling, what they were revealing about how my bodily systems were interacting with each other. For the first time in my life, they were starting to make sense. I was connecting the dots and working on each part of my body, each system, with a new level of clarity.

As I began to see how systems-thinking applied so much more effectively to understanding and managing menopause, compared to the traditional compartmentalized symptoms-treatment, I knew at an incredibly deep level that I had to become formally educated to finish putting it all together and open the door to my healing. So, in June 2022, four months after my surgical menopause, I went back to school in this field. I attended the MindBodyFood Institute and became a certified women's holistic hormone health practitioner.

While I had started writing about my journey (the genesis of this book) very early on, once I was armed with my formal education, I felt there was more to share with the world. I decided to do a podcast to share my story. As I worked with my podcast producer, he began to push me on my message and what I wanted to be known for. The fuzziness lifted. I wanted to give hope to women, but I also wanted to help them find their way back to healing. A book and podcast, while great, were not going to be enough. I wanted actual coaches available to provide women with individual solutions. So I put a team together. During my hormone practitioner certification program, I had met with the most experienced hormone practitioners. I reached out to them with my coaching concept; they loved it. I then met with doctors who were systems thinkers who agreed to help the women we would educate. And from there, Meno Coaching was born. The more my purpose got clear, the more freedom I felt. My healing came not from pushing back but from finding a way to turn my pain into purpose. In creating this service for women, I was reminded of how big God is. In all of my pain, I had forgotten. This was proof that He is bigger and more able than I ever realized.

Meno Coaching (menocoaching.com) is now live with lab testing, coaching support, and a doctor referral network. We have already worked with many women to help them understand their bodies, to become educated, and to become their own advocates. We have helped women with PMS, PMDD, PCOS, perimenopause, menopause, and surgical menopause. The most effective way to solve the puzzle of our healing is to accumulate, assemble, and analyze the data that we receive through lab testing. Thus, we guide each client toward the best available and most appropriate lab tests to assess *all* of their affected body systems, not just one. Following are the lab tests that were most critical for my healing and that our entire team highly recommends to clients.

Comprehensive CBC (Complete Blood Count) Panel

This common blood panel offers an important picture of overall health that includes identifying and counting white blood cells, red blood cells, and platelets and helps to determine if there are other underlying medical conditions like inflammation, infection, or immune disorder. The CBC panel is the first piece of the puzzle.

DUTCH Complete™ Test

The hormone ratio between estrogen and progesterone is key to balancing the entire endocrine system. Measuring our hormone levels is important, but just as important is understanding how we metabolize those hormones during perimenopause, menopause, and surgical menopause. Why? Because the way each of us metabolizes hormones is different and is impacted by our liver, gut, adrenal glands, stress, and nutrition. Understanding our individual hormone metabolism as well as their ratios is *essential* for optimal health and healing.

The DUTCH Complete™ Test measures sex hormone amounts as well as how we use and detoxify these hormones. It also identifies free cortisol versus bound cortisol. Free cortisol is active and able to give energy and, at the right amount, decrease inflammation. Bound cortisol is inactive and lacks the ability to impact the body. We need this to know how much of each we have to effectively manage our healing journey. The DUTCH Complete™ measures estrogen, testosterone, progesterone, and adrenals as well as B6, B12, glutathione, dopamine, epinephrine, and melatonin. It is a truly comprehensive guide to understanding how to manage root cause symptoms. It taught me what I needed to know to advocate for myself. Today, I provide this to my menopausal clients as their second puzzle piece. I suggest not getting additional tests until they have completed this test first and received some sound consulting about the information it provides.

Mira Fertility Tracker and App

During perimenopause, progesterone drops and estrogen seesaws up and down. It's unpredictable, which, historically, made it difficult to find enough of a trend to understand when one needs supplements or hormone therapy. However, with the advent of fertility trackers, women can now track their hormone fluctuations. The Mira fertility tracker (miracare.com) offers women lab-grade technology to measure levels of multiple hormones at home. And it offers an app that automatically tracks and analyzes hormone patterns. For women in perimenopause, this allows them to track their cycles and hormone levels in order to hone in on trends that can help them determine how close to or far they are from menopause. Or, if they've already reached menopause, the tracker and app helps them find their sweet spot in hormone therapy. My experience using Mira is nothing short of incredible and something I wish I would have known about during perimenopause.

GI-MAP™ for Gut Health

The gut has an enormous impact on neurotransmitters and our body's ability to detoxify environmental toxins and hormones. When the gut is not balanced, hormones are not balanced, and the brain also suffers. Poor gut health increases the chances of inflammation, PCOS, endometriosis, and breast cancer. The GI-MAP™, in my opinion, is the best test for understanding gut health because it looks at bacterial pathogens, parasitic pathogens, and viral pathogens. Our team looks at the data and uses the results to guide women to nutritional and supplemental support to clean up the gut.

I saw immediate changes in my mood, energy, and overall digestion after cleaning up several gut issues, including an overgrowth of yeast and even, at one point, E. coli. I also found out that my body was unable to absorb fats or nutrients appropriately. Sometimes, we may eat the right food, but our bodies are not effectively absorbing the nutrients and micronutrients from that food. This knowledge drastically impacted my ability to heal as supplementing digestive enzymes allowed my body to receive energy again from my food!

NutrEval® Profile

Most of us try but don't get all the nutrition we need due to poor eating habits. Nutrients are keys that unlock our brain power, our energy, our gut health, and many other physiological processes. The NutrEval® Profile looks at 125 biomarkers and assesses antioxidants, vitamins, minerals, essential fatty acids, amino acids, and digestive nutrients. It is the motherload of all panels on nutrition. It is vital that we understand where our body needs support. It also helps to know not just how to supplement, but how to fuel our body through sound nutrition, which means less sugar, less processed food, and the removal of trans fats and xenoestrogens from our diet and lifestyle as much as possible. Xenoestrogens are compounds found in plastics and chemicals in our homes that mimic estrogen and contribute to many of the health issues we see today. I knew very little about this until my own healing journey.

Full Thyroid Panel

The thyroid hormones, in particular T3, T4, and Reverse T3, are the masters of all hormones. They have a substantial impact on mood, weight, and estrogen metabolism. Rarely do doctors test all necessary aspects of these critical hormones. I have learned the following through my own experience: TSH (thyroid stimulating hormone), which is produced by the pituitary gland, indicates how much thyroid hormone is bound and how much is circulating in the body. The level of free T3 tells how much of the most potent part of the hormone is active to impact a positive mood, weight, and energy. Free T4 reveals how much of the inactive hormone someone has and if it is converting to T3 or not. Last is Reverse T3, and this one is very interesting. We can have high T3 and still feel heavy, bloated, sluggish, foggy, depressed, muscle pain, and otherwise unwell. Reverse T3 shows whether the body is effectively utilizing T3. If not, we are likely deficient and need supplementation through a doctor's care. If things look abnormal, we will need an antibody test to make sure we do not have Hashimoto's, which is an autoimmune disorder of the thyroid gland. Push for this test; recovery depends on it. For more information, visit StoptheThyroidMadness.com.

Navigating the Healing: My Map

Resilience is a requirement for survival in surgical menopause. I was told I would feel fine three months post surgery. Medical professionals said the patch would take over, and everything would be normal. But my friends who had experienced surgical menopause said it would take a year for me to feel like myself again. It did. There's no magic bullet to healing from surgical menopause. It's like peeling back layers of an onion and requires a woman to find the grit that only comes from very deep within. Every woman has to be willing to learn and utilize the science and unearth the data that will work for her. While a worthy and necessary investment in oneself, it's a process that takes time. I spent months tweaking, testing, and adjusting before I found what worked best for my body. The process itself was exhausting and left me feeling like my whole life was being lived around symptoms, journaling, and just trying to survive each day.

But I was convinced I could heal my own body through my ability to balance myself based on my symptoms, the guidance of good lab tests, and my personal resilience and faith. I had uncovered all the key pieces of the puzzle; it was time to put them to work. I had a destination and had decided to take responsibility to navigate my journey. I just needed a map. So I made one.

My map to healing included three components: body, mind, and spirit. I am convinced that all three must be aligned for anyone to become fully healthy and whole. This is true not only for the menopausal woman who is suffering, but for anyone suffering from any ailment. I remain firm in this belief because we were created by the Creator for all three of these complex pieces to work in complete harmony. "You see, you are a spirit, you have a soul and you live in a body. You have emotions, you have thoughts, you have a will, and you have a conscience. You are a complex being! And Jesus came to heal every single part of you. There's not one part that He doesn't want to make completely whole" (Meyer).

We are not one-size-fits-all during this transition. Too often, we are viewed by physicians as if we are like every other patient they see, so we are treated as such. This could not be more flawed! It is why we must navigate our own healing journey.

Below is *my* map, the steps I took to find balance and total healing. I offer it as a guide, as food for thought for anyone else designing their own map for their own journey to healing.

The Body

The body is incredibly complex. Science has provided advanced insights into how we are wired and what our bodies need to thrive and feel alive. There are very basic needs that must be met to find this energy. As simple as it may sound, we have forgotten their impact.

Hormones

Finding hormonal balance is obviously critical to the perimenopausal and menopausal woman. Being on estrogen, progesterone, testosterone, thyroid, and DHEA at the right doses have brought my body, mind, and spirit healing, but it was a long and arduous journey to reach that balance.

Carrying the ESR1 gene mutation made my navigation into menopause very difficult. Being ultra sensitive to estrogen made it hard to find balance. For me, it was just as important to find the right amount of estrogen as to manage my sensitivity through how I metabolized it. I used my Mira app to monitor my levels and symptoms, which allowed me to manage hormone dosages.

For the first three months after surgery, I was on a 0.01 mg patch. It was an inexpensive generic patch and covered by insurance. At first, I felt great, no problems, like it would be smooth sailing. Then, the fluctuations started all over again. Thankfully, after three months of ups and downs, Dr. M. suggested a change to a name-brand patch. She said my sensitivity might reject the chemical make-up of the generic patch because it had fillers which might have impacted how I was feeling. I also experienced significant bloating, and my legs and ankles looked like swollen logs. So, in addition to switching to a name-brand patch, we lowered the dose. But it was a battle with the insurance company for approval for the name-brand patch. Dr. M. fought for me and wrote a novel to the insurance company on why my body needed something "cleaner." God help us. She was brilliant. We also had to work on my progesterone dosage to ensure that my estrogen to progesterone ratio was balanced.

The new patch felt much better, but then my body realized my estrogen levels had dropped, and my anxiety and OCD came back with a vengeance. I couldn't win. I decided I needed to stick it out, to give it time. The women on the Facebook Surmeno Connection page said it likely would take four to six weeks for my body to adapt to any change. Sure enough, after a period of four weeks, I felt much more stable. For the first three months after we lowered the dosage, as my body adjusted, I tested my estrogen levels everyday using the Mira app and journaled both my symptoms and levels each day. Journaling was critical to understanding what was happening in my body. I finally started to have better days until another part of my system decided it was tired: my thyroid. One thing impacts another.

Thyroid Gland

I had no idea (because nobody told me) that BHRT, particularly estrogen replacement therapy, can negatively impact the thyroid gland in women who suffer from hypothyroidism, like me. Estrogen therapy can increase certain transport proteins that then need more thyroid hormone than the thyroid can produce (Kjaergaard et al. Introduction). In effect, estrogen therapy can impact thyroid function. A dysfunction of the thyroid gland can cause fatigue, constipation, muscle aches, and, for some, even depression. I became constipated, and my legs felt like bricks. I had pain everywhere; I thought I was sick. I told my endocrinologist that something was wrong, and that I suspected my thyroid. (I was starting to become my own doctor.) So, we tested it. Turns out, my T3 was stable but my Reverse T3 had tripled since surgery. I know this was my body's way of trying to reserve my energy as it healed and shunted all my energy to survival. We also tested my iron level; it had dropped by more than half since the surgery. Iron impacts thyroid … the pieces fit. My doctor suggested T3 only, but we both underestimated the ability of my adrenal glands to keep up. I was so jittery and shaky that I couldn't walk. My body could not tolerate the stimulation of the straight T3. Thankfully, I knew what was happening and lowered my dose. My DO also recommended that I take selenium to help convert my T4 to T3 naturally as another way to avoid taking large amounts of T3. It took a week to calm down. I became very good at knowing when too much was too much and how to ask my doctors to test to get what I needed.

Iron

Though I lowered my T3 dose, my body still struggled to tolerate it because my adrenal glands were not strong enough, and my slow COMT gene was recirculating too many neurotransmitters, thus causing anxiety. I needed to go low and slow and support my sluggish adrenal system that I'd taken advantage of for years. I went back to the basics of adrenal support and started to take extra vitamin C, magnesium, and vitamin B6 P5P to support my slow COMT mutation. I also asked the women on the Surmeno Connection page about the iron. Turns out, my months of fatigue were largely from low iron. Many women on the site had experienced the same. I still cannot understand why no medical professional had proactively let me know that surgery can lower iron stores and that it takes up to six months to come back without supplementation! I started on adrenal powder support and a liquid iron so that I would not become constipated, and, within five weeks, I felt a huge change. I felt like parts of me were finally waking up.

Movement

If we don't move and poop enough, estrogen will recirculate in our body. It sounds gross, but it is a fact, and, unless we detoxify through these two methods, we could end up with estrogen dominance. Yes, even with no ovaries and BHRT! Beyond its importance to healthy estrogen levels, movement increases natural serotonin and dopamine levels, which help women feel peaceful and happy. It has been proven that forty-five minutes of walking very briskly has the same effect as taking an antidepressant but with zero side effects.

As I healed after surgery, it became clear that my body could no longer tolerate "hard core" intense workouts. I'd be exhausted for twenty-four hours if I pushed too hard. While I wanted to push myself because the high of exercise gave me temporary relief from my anxiety, my adrenal glands could no longer tolerate it. So, I listened to my body and changed my approach. I became a student of yoga and the benefits of stretching and breathing. I started Pilates and walked three miles a day. My body wanted to move but not to be driven to a cortisol marathon. As I stood facing myself in the mirror during a yoga practice, I saw someone different. I saw someone strong and at peace. I saw my inner warrior. Not striving, just standing in faith grounded in who I was for the first time in a year, maybe the first time in my whole life. My stress levels decreased, and I learned the power of breathing through my yoga practice. Breathing gives life, reduces stress, and detoxifies our bodies. Movement with breathing is healing. When we first arrived on Earth, God breathed life into us. It is this same breath that can sustain us when we need to find our center. It's there all day, ready to access. This has been invaluable to me.

Nutrition

Lets face it, everything we do in life is connected to eating. We celebrate with food, we socialize with friends at restaurants, and we sometimes even self-medicate with food. It is tied to our survival, but what we ingest often eats at us in more ways than one.

Processed sugary foods wreak havoc on our bodies and increase inflammation in our gut and entire endocrine system. We have replaced nutrient-dense food with anything that tastes gooey, greasy, cheesy, and sweet. Studies show that companies actually promote these foods because they trigger the pleasure center of our brain when consumed. Yup, dopamine!! It's no surprise we are addicted to the things that are the worst for our bodies. We fall into the trap of eating to feel pleasure versus eating to fuel our cells.

Consequently, we often lack key nutrients critical to our healing. But the only way to know where we stand is to get sound data on our nutrients. I took the NutrEval® Profile nutrition assessment when I started menopause. It showed that my blood sugar was very unstable during menopause, which is common, and that I needed to eat smaller amounts of food more regularly. I also realized that I had stopped eating some of the most basic foods needed for my healing. So, I dramatically changed my food choices and the amounts I ate. I believe with my whole heart that food is medicine. I increased my intake of fresh organic greens, particularly cruciferous vegetables. I started eating berries every day at breakfast. I added in eggs for protein three times a week as well as more fish and other lean meats. Quinoa became a major staple as I needed the fiber to keep my estrogen levels balanced. I had nuts for a snack and began drinking water with lemon all day long. I cut down coffee to half a cup a day and added green tea in the afternoon. I actually looked forward to shopping for healthy options and made better choices. The changes to my body composition and energy levels were dramatic. My skin was even better, and, overall, I felt lighter but stronger. My system was getting the fuel it so desperately needed to feel energized. It has been life changing, and I am at my ideal weight, even through menopause. I continue to take the NutrEval® Profile every six to eight months. The information is invaluable in helping me to better understand any deficiencies that may arise.

The Gut

The gut is known by many as the second brain. "The gut-brain axis (GBA) consists of bidirectional communication between the central and the enteric nervous system, linking emotional and cognitive centers of the brain with peripheral intestinal functions. Recent advances in research have described the importance of gut microbiota in influencing these reactions" (Carabotti et al. Abstract). My gut was a mess. I had too much bad bacteria and not enough good bacteria to help my brain to function properly. After extensive gut testing, I started a high-fiber diet, probiotics with plenty of the strains that my tests suggested I needed, and prebiotics. I also started digestive enzymes to help me to digest food, another piece to my complex puzzle. In just thirty days, my stool was regular, soft, and consistent. After years of constipation, I finally felt light and healthy. All of that bad bacteria was literally from years of rotting stool; worse, that bad bacteria was impacting my ability to clear my estrogen. I was finally able to take out the trash!!

Sleep

Sleep is an absolute must to finding healing and balance in the body. It is the only time the body can truly repair itself and reboot. During sleep, cortisol and insulin are at their lowest points, which enables the body to break down fat. A lack of sleep can easily cause hormone imbalances and, hence, cause us to become irritable, fatigued, and gain weight. During perimenopause, I began to wake up a lot at night, which really drained my energy during the day. I investigated ways to get not just more sleep but deeper sleep. I found that taking 500 mg of magnesium an hour before bed would settle my body and mind. It was life changing. I also took my progesterone before bed, which increased my GABA and calmed me down. I drank chamomile tea and committed to kicking technology out of my bedroom at 8:30 pm. I learned how to dial down so my body could recognize a pattern of rest and restoration. Falling asleep at the same time each day and waking at the same time is very important to the circadian rhythm, as is getting sunlight every morning for twenty minutes, which has been proven to increase deeper sleep at night. I started going to bed by 10:00 pm every night and noticed that my body naturally awoke at 6:30 am. My new regimen gave me deeper levels of sleep and more daytime energy. I noticed within only five short weeks that I was no longer waking up more than once at night. I was truly getting restorative sleep, and it felt so good!!

Supplements

I could write an entire book on supplementation!! In fact, I would describe myself as a biohacker. "Biohacking, also known as human augmentation or human enhancement, is do-it-yourself biology aimed at improving performance, health, and wellbeing through strategic interventions" (Marr). I take many different kinds of supplements for different deficiencies based on my nutrient panel results. Here, I will highlight the ones that I believe are most critical for a woman going through menopause.

> **Vitamin C:** Critical for the repair of all body tissues, the formation of collagen, the absorption of iron, and a strong immune system. Protects against free radicals and supports the adrenals.
>
> **Vitamin B6:** Important for the brain and the nervous system. Turns food into energy. Synthesizes neurotransmitters.
>
> **Vitamin B12:** Helps with cell formation and bone health, improves mood and depression, and, overall, energizes the body and mind.
>
> **Vitamin D3:** Strengthens the immune system, enhances mood, and regulates insulin levels.
>
> **Zinc Picolinate:** Acts as an antioxidant and protects cells against damage. Incredibly important for immune function and testosterone metabolism.
>
> **Glutathione:** Plays a crucial role in immune function and detoxification and lowers inflammation.
>
> **Methylfolate:** Effective for helping with depression and regulating mood and other brain functions (this must be supported with careful guidance due to gene mutations).
>
> **Magnesium:** Impacts over eight hundred chemical processes in the body, including energy production, cortisol, calmness, and cell metabolism.

I have found that these supplements have enhanced my hormone therapy while also providing me with greater clarity, energy, and a positive mood. They have also been key to my detoxification of estrogen to keep my systems healthy and balanced and key to my brain health and emotional balance. Managing the process of supplementation takes work. It should only be done under a doctor's care with nutritional testing that is both thorough and accurate. Even though these are supplements, they still change the body's chemistry! Based on my own history of chemical sensitivity, I always tell clients that the "low and slow" method is best. I also encourage them not to try too many at once, or they will not know what is or is not working. Supplements never take the place of good nutrition.

The Mind

I regularly tell my clients that the thing between their ears is the most important tool to healing and wholeness. Despite the fact that we often conflate them, the mind is different from the brain. According to Caroline Leaf, "The most fundamental definition of your mind is how you think, feel, and choose. The mind works through the brain: the brain is the physical organ that filters and responds to the mind" (53). The brain is the organ and the mind is where we have the information and power to impact the brain. This is where God and science are interconnected. Romans 12:2 says, "Be transformed by the renewing of your mind." It was always God's plan that we use our mind to change our brain and even our body's ability to heal. Every cell responds to our thoughts. Chemicals change, hormones change, digestion can increase or slow—all because of our thoughts. Unfortunately, more often than not, we let our thoughts lead us. I always struggled with that. In many ways, my anxiety was like a runaway train of my thoughts. Unpacking this was key to my freedom from suffering and, more importantly, was the gateway to healing my body. How we think is incredibly powerful and can rob us or give us life. Dr. Leaf's deep research proved this: "As we think, the brain literally changes in hundreds of thousands of ways on cellular, molecular, chemical, genetic, and structural levels. More research is being published on a daily basis showing how every functional, chemical, and physical feature on the brain can be and is transformed as we use our mind. The key is you can direct this process" (55).

I had gone to work on my body; it was time to work on my mind. Science has proven that through neuroplasticity we can change our brain wiring. Mindful focus on redirecting our thoughts changes our biochemistry; it causes new neurons to form. It took years to create the thoughts that I carried with me into menopause. They were formed from my experiences, my pain, and every agreement I'd made with myself to survive through it all. Changing them would take regular committed practice. But I was unwilling to leave that work undone. With my history of OCD, I often wondered if I could learn to combat my thoughts. I had been given a label, and even that had impacted the way I viewed myself. I decided *no more labels*. The only label that mattered, that would sit over me, would be that I was a child of God. Righteous because of His sacrifice for me. It was time to stop believing lies and cling to what I knew was true.

Grounding myself in the truth became my cornerstone when my body signals were misfiring and I was riding the roller coaster of my hormones. My mind was truly the battlefield. My commitment to managing my mind was a daily activity that required work and focus. I started each day with prayer and reading the Word of God, which for me is truth. Writing down my thoughts, reflecting and addressing these thoughts and their roots, and choosing to believe facts versus feelings were very important to my healing. I noticed what triggered my ruminations, and, when I was triggered, I went deeper to understand why I was so shaken. When I looked, I found answers. Most of them were in the wounds of my past. Being rejected and abandoned by the people who were supposed to love me the most developed a defensiveness in my heart and a strong desire to protect myself because I had believed that nobody ever protected me. But I was wrong. God protected me. He was in every moment of my life. He never left. I was still here, and now I had something to say. He was pulling up weeds and making beauty from ash.

During the transition of menopause, I had to face myself. I realized through it all that nothing, absolutely nothing, would have stopped me from driving too hard except surgical menopause. This was where my belief in something much bigger than myself made me realize there is a grand plan for my life and for the life of each one of us. If I didn't learn the lesson, I would walk the forty-year journey of learning instead of the eleven-day journey. I had to learn how to *rest—* mentally as well as physically. "Rest" was always a dirty word for me until I realized that my lack of it was actually making me less effective at work, not more effective. And my inability to rest was making deep intimacy in my life less likely. I was always on to the next thing. With surgical menopause, I realized I could no longer push through as I had done for years. It stopped me dead in my tracks.

Lifestyle/Stress Management

Stress is a driver of performance. We need stress to focus and raise adrenaline to execute our goals. *Dis*tress is when stress is out of balance in our lives. This kind of stress is what causes cortisol release, inflammation, weight gain, and even heart attacks or strokes. I never was "tuned in" to my stress levels. In fact, I believed in my core that more stress meant greater output. That's true to a degree, but chronic stress leads to imbalance and inflammation in the body and even in the brain. During menopause, we have less reserves as all of our body's resources are being utilized to fight the endless ups and downs of the biological changes. Therefore, our ability to learn how to manage stress and become resilient is crucial to our sustainable health and healing. Unfortunately, our society encourages working and stressing more, not less, and few medical professionals talk about developing tools for greater resilience.

I had no idea how much I would need to re-evaluate my life and my stress levels during menopause. I had to rewire my brain. Everything I had learned about what success looked like needed to be reviewed. I started with sleep as my first priority. My hard-working Energizer bunny self was now like a computer faced with a total force quit. But it was necessary, and it was healing. I sleep eight hours minimum per night, and it feels wonderful.

Next was work. My job had always been my master. For many years, I believed that I truly lived to work. It was hard to admit that even when one's work is serving and helping others, it can become a master in a way God never intended. To lower my stress, I had to choose to use my gifts in a way that was deliberate and life giving, and I had to say no when my schedule was getting too hectic. I hated this, and sometimes still do, but it was necessary. As a bonus, the quality of my work went up three times what it was before. My ability to take care of myself was providing care for others. My approach to my own life and my ability to find a healthy balance was positively impacting my clients. I had lived a life of being led by my work rather than leading it within a bigger framework of my purpose. I say no now without guilt; I work four days a week; and I am finished with work by 4:30 pm each day. My work performance has gone up, and I am much happier. Trust me, there is something here to learn.

In the middle of the upheaval of menopause in all its forms, we desperately need our minds to listen to our bodies' need for balance, to hear the whispers. We need to revisit how we manage stress and how to become resilient. This is the intersection of body, mind, and emotions. We are all of these things, and each one impacts the other two. We have to listen to where we feel the stress and "talk back" to it. I think of it as PAC-MAN. We only have so many energy bars per day (much less during "the change"), and we need to decide each day how to spend that energy. Managing mental and physical energy is essential to healing and wholeness.

The Spirit

We are all a Spirit. We have a soul, and we live in a body. The Spirit is where Christians believe we hear from God. It is our conscience. Our soul is our mind, our will, and our emotions. The body is the house we live in. During menopause, my flesh became very weak and my emotions became very hard to control. Then there was that bathroom floor. I screamed on that floor; I cried on that floor; and it was there where I would get counsel in my spirit from God. It was my threshing floor, the place where my transformation was happening. The separation of the good from the bad. I felt so helpless some days, but, as much as I hurt, God never left. Sometimes it was an hour, sometimes thirty minutes. I would lift my head off the floor, and He would release me from the oppression. No matter how much we research and educate ourselves, there is no substitute for God's holy power in our life. God is the ultimate healer and physician.

I believe with my whole heart that there is a place where only God can enter for our healing. A place where the Spirit and its power is the only force that can help us while we struggle to find ourselves in the transition. I was so weak in my mind, emotions, and body that I decided to double down on my Spirit to find my peace and a foundation I could cling to. Thank God for His Holy Spirit inside me! I held onto it like oxygen; it was my life raft. In our lives, God can guide our decisions, carry our heavy burdens, and bring us peace, even in the middle of the struggle.

The What and the Why Collide

As I began to experience healing in my body, my purpose surfaced. My relentless pursuit to find answers and help others drove me to a place of understanding how God wanted to use my pain for good. I got more traction the more I guided clients through their own painful experiences and realized that without my own experience, I would have no compassion for these women. I realized that while we blame doctors for not having all the answers, we must also be our own answer. We must learn to listen to our bodies' whispers and give them what they require before they scream. We need to stop ignoring the messages we receive; we need to awaken to what we are hearing in our souls. It is not a quick fix. There is, however, a way to find out what our body needs and bring the system to homeostasis.

As I was finishing this book, I got COVID, and I got it bad. I was in the hospital on a drip. My body, once again, felt like it was depleted after I had finally found my way out of my hormone madness. I got depressed and felt moments of anxiety. I wanted to stop suffering. After surviving COVID, I was in a horrible accident that caused two disk bulges in my neck, another major setback. I then found out that the person who hit me died. I crumbled on that bathroom floor again. As if the suffering was not already enough, my dad died suddenly four days after my car accident. Remember at the beginning of this book I wrote about us having an Enemy? This was further proof. It was clear that I was fighting a spiritual battle.

Then, something happened. The second miracle in my life. I felt a very powerful welling inside of me. A clear, spiritual welling of God's power. I was a conqueror through Him. I would fight this. God was my Redeemer. I was going to tell the world my story even if it killed me. I knew from a very young age that I was going to make a difference, an impact. I knew I had gifts to serve and help others. Earlier in my life, I misused those gifts to make myself feel important. Over the last decade, I finally realized that the work being done on me through this hell was to transform me from the inside out. My gifts never left me, but now they are servant-led and have nothing to do with me and everything to do with God's perfect plan for my life. My brokenness had to happen to bring me to a place of surrender and dedication to a higher calling. I've proclaimed obedience to the One who called me to Himself no matter what the cost. I decided that I wanted to be faithful, not famous. That was my true calling. Today, I am blessed to work with women who sound much like I did. They are stuck, they have no hope, and they feel that the system has failed them. We provide not only coaching and lab testing, but proof with hope that they can thrive again, even transform.

The menopause "why" is about *transformation*; that is its ultimate purpose. I can tell you with full honesty that I am no longer who I was. Some pieces broke off and died through all of this. Others bloomed and grew and brought sunlight. For anything to grow, we need to pull out the weeds. The flowers will not bloom without the work. I have done the work. I have tilled my soil, and there is freedom in it.

The Purpose

As I reflect on everything that has happened and the severity of it all, I realize one truth. Without all of this struggle and suffering, three things would have never happened. First, I would never have known God this intimately and profoundly. Second, I would never have become the person He wanted me to become. Third, the gifts I was given would have been distorted, misused, and all about me instead of about Him and in service to others. That was my purpose in menopause. The brokenness had to happen to revive my heart and soul, to find my way home to the girl who loved to sing and held so much compassion. She is back, and she is much better equipped to live a life of service and love. All the covering up is gone. I was put through the struggle, refined by the fire, molded by the Potter's hands, and He turned my pain into purpose, my brokenness into beauty.

There is a true purpose in the menopause transition. Just like puberty, marriage, birth, and death are rites of passage, so is menopause. There is no surprise that it comes in the final chapter of life, the last half. It is so that we can heal our bodies, heal our hurts, and find our soul, our voice, and our purpose. Some embrace the change. Others, like me, push back, wanting to be who we once were. I can say with my whole heart that, after menopause, we are no longer who we were, nor are we meant to be that person anymore. We have been created to evolve through the last chapter by being different and *better* than we were.

May you strive to find healing for yourself. May you feel comfort in the struggle as you know it's moving you to a life filled with joy and the ability to thrive. Most importantly, may you know through these words that it *is* possible.

Works Cited

Almey, Anne, et al. "Estrogen receptors in the central nervous system and their implication for dopamine-dependent cognition in females." *Hormones and Behavior*, vol. 74, Aug. 2015, pp. 125–138.

Attwells, Sophia, et al. "Inflammation in the Neurocircuitry of Obsessive-Compulsive Disorder." *JAMA Psychiatry*, vol. 74, no. 8, 1 Aug. 2017, pp. 833–840.

Bluming, Avrum, and Carol Tavris. *Estrogen Matters*. Little, Brown Spark, 2018.

Brighten, Jolene. "Guide to Treating PMDD." *Menstrual Cycle*, 2 Sept. 2021, drbrighten.com/guide-to-treating-pmdd-premenstrual-dysphoric-disorder. Accessed 25 July 2023.

Carabotti, Marilia, et al. "The gut-brain axis: interactions between enteric microbiota, central and enteric nervous systems." *Annals of Gastroenterology*, vol. 28, no. 2, Apr.–June 2015, pp. 203–209.

Cleveland Clinic. "Perimenopause." *Cleveland Clinic Health Library*, 5 Oct. 2021, my.clevelandclinic.org/health/diseases/21608-perimenopause. Accessed 12 June 2023.

Cloud, Henry, and John Townsend. *How People Grow*. Zondervan, 2001.

Englert-Golan, Monika, et al. "Altered Expression of *ESR1*, *ESR2*, *PELP1* and *c-SRC* Genes Is Associated with Ovarian Cancer Manifestation." *International Journal of Molecular Sciences*, vol. 22, no. 12, 9 June 2021, 6216.

Gaspar, Joana. "Is polycystic ovary syndrome a hypothalamic disease?" *eBioMedicine*, vol. 92, 29 Apr. 2023, 104598, doi.org/10.1016/j.ebiom.2023.104598. Accessed 26 July 2023.

Gersh, Felice. "Why I'm One OB/GYN Who Is Not Prescribing the Birth Control Pill." *The ZRT Laboratory Blog*, 1 Nov. 2018, zrtlab.com/blog/archive/obgyn-not-prescribing-the-birth-control-pill. Accessed 12 June 2023.

Greenberg, Melanie. "Understanding the Trauma Brain." *Psychology Today*, 30 June 2021, psychologytoday.com/us/blog/the-mindful-self-express/202106/understanding-the-trauma-brain. Accessed 8 June 2023.

Hawkins, Amy Lee. *What You Must Know About Bioidentical Hormone Replacement Therapy*. Square One Publishers, 2013.

Hwang, Wu Jeong, et al. "The Role of Estrogen Receptors and Their Signaling across Psychiatric Disorders." *International Journal of Molecular Sciences*, vol. 22, no. 1, 2021, 373.

Institute for Functional Medicine. "What is Functional Medicine?" Homepage, 2023, ifm.org. Accessed 27 July 2023.

Johansson, Asa, et al. "Investigating the Effect of Estradiol Levels on the Risk of Breast, Endometrial, and Ovarian Cancer." *Journal of the Endocrine Society*, vol. 6, no. 8, 1 Aug. 2022, bvac100.

Kjaergaard, Alisa, et al. "Thyroid function, sex hormones and sexual function: a Mendelian randomization study." *European Journal of Epidemiology*, vol. 36, 6 Feb. 2021, pp. 335–344.

Kulkarni, Jayashri, et al. "The prevalence of early life trauma in premenstrual dysphoric disorder (PMDD)." *Psychiatry Research*, vol. 308, Feb. 2022, 114381.

Leaf, Caroline. *Cleaning Up Your Mental Mess*. Baker Books, 2021.

Lynch, Ben. *Dirty Genes*. HarperOne, 2018.

Marr, Bernard. "What's Biohacking? All You Need To Know About The Latest Health Craze." *Forbes*, 26 Feb. 2021, forbes.com/sites/ bernardmarr/2021/02/26/whats-biohacking-all-you-need-to-know- about-the-latest-health-craze. Accessed 15 June 2023.

Meyer, Joyce. "Joyce Meyer Quotes." *BrainyQuote.com*, brainyquote. com/quotes/joyce_meyer_567640. Accessed 15 June 2023.

MedlinePlus: National Library of Medicine. "Can genes be turned on and off in cells?" *How Genes Work*, 26 Mar. 2021, medlineplus. gov/genetics/understanding/howgeneswork/geneonoff. Accessed 31 July 2023.

Northrup, Christiane. *The Wisdom of Menopause*. Bantam Books, 2021.

Orloff, Judith. *The Empath's Survival Guide*. Sounds True, 2018.

RN Labs. "Methylation & Mental Health: An Introduction." *Methylation and Genetics: Blog*, 12 Jan. 2016, rnlabs.com.au/ methylation-an-introduction. Accessed 31 July 2023.

Schwartz, Jeffrey, and Sharon Begley. *The Mind and the Brain*. Regan Books, 2003.

Senge, Peter. *The Fifth Discipline*. Currency, 2006.

Van der Kolk, Bessel. *The Body Keeps the Score*. Viking Penguin, 2014.

Weinberg, Jennifer. "The Estrobolome." *Simple Pure Whole Wellness*, 25 Sept. 2019, jenniferweinbergmd.com/estrobolome. Accessed 12 June 2023.

About the Author

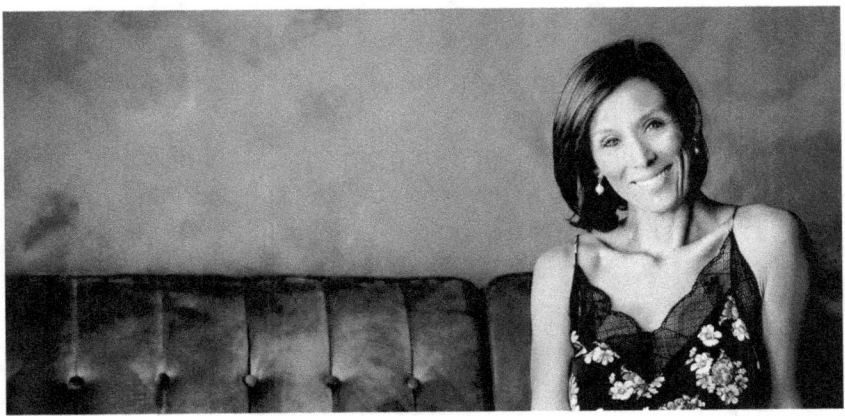

Irene Ortiz-Glass, founder and CEO of Leadership Advisory Group, LLC, and founder of Meno Coaching, is a twenty-year executive, coach, and consultant who has dedicated her career to helping people find purpose, healing, and joy.

After over a decade of global talent management and general management experience, Irene founded Leadership Advisory Group. The organization is committed to helping executives thrive in work and life. With extensive experience helping individual leaders suffering from burnout, perfectionism, and overachievement, her coaching moves beyond the usual business strategies and guides them in self-reflection and self-improvement. The intention with her clients is to reach a holistic integration of professional achievement and personal growth in order to create a life of significance. Additionally, she collaborates with executive teams to facilitate strategic planning, organizational development, change management, and goal alignment through a comprehensive organization-wide framework that fosters a shared sense of purpose and unity. Irene is especially dedicated to nurturing high-potential women leaders, including annually sponsoring the Women in Leadership initiative to equip women with the confidence and skills to reach their potential and thrive in life.

An author, speaker, and outspoken women's advocate, Irene is passionate about helping women cultivate a fulfilling life—physically, mentally, emotionally, and spiritually. After experiencing years of PMS, a difficult journey through a decade of perimenopause, and, ultimately, surgical menopause, Irene decided to take her health into her own hands and became a certified hormone practitioner. From there, she launched Meno Coaching, a team of experts who provide end-to-end support for women throughout the complex journey of perimenopause and menopause. Through education, lab testing, coaching support, and access to a valuable physician network of vetted menopause specialists, Irene and her team help women to become their own advocate and guide them on a path to healing. She also hosts the "What I Wish I Knew: Beyond Menopause" podcast, which is dedicated to helping women thrive through the menopausal transition. A woman of faith who believes with God all things are possible, Irene cares deeply about wellness, nutrition, spirit-filled living, and finding purpose.

Irene has a bachelor's degree in communications from Azusa Pacific University, a master's degree in organizational leadership from Chapman University, and is certified as a women's holistic hormone health practitioner through the MindBodyFood Institute.

To connect with Irene and learn more about her work, please visit leadershipadvisorygroup.com and menocoaching.com.